# COMMUNICABLE
# DISEASE
# HANDBOOK

# COMMUNICABLE DISEASE HANDBOOK

**L. Claire Bennett, B.S.N.** • **Sarah Searl, M.S.**

University of British Columbia
School of Nursing
Vancouver, British Columbia

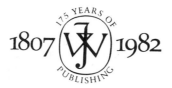

1807 1982

A WILEY MEDICAL PUBLICATION
**JOHN WILEY & SONS**
**New York • Chichester • Brisbane • Toronto •**
**Singapore**

*Cover design: Wanda Lubelska*
*Production: Audrey Pavey*

**Library of Congress Cataloging in Publication Data:**

Bennett, L. Claire.
  Communicable disease handbook.

  (A Wiley medical publication)
  Includes index.
    1. Communicable diseases.   2. Communicable diseases—
Preventive inoculation.   3. Epidemiology.   I. Searl,
Sarah.   II. Title.   III. Series.   [DNLM:   1. Communicable
diseases—Handbooks.   WC 100 B471c]
RA643.B46   1983        614.4        82-11062
ISBN 0-471-09271-1

Printed in the United States of America

10 9 8 7 6 5 4 3 2 1

# Preface

How often have you scanned a variety of references, searching for information on a contagious disease or an immunization rationale? If you do uncover the condition, why is the related health teaching so often ignored?

You probably wondered, as we did, why these conditions regularly encountered in the practice of community health had not been dealt with more succinctly.

This handbook answers those questions. It is a ready reference for health sciences students and professionals serving the community as they encounter the public's health concerns. Occupational health and medical office nurses will find the handbook a useful tool in counseling clients. Allied health team members, such as dentists and nutritionists, can also use the information on health teaching in their work with families. The handbook is organized to promote self-directed study by setting out content areas, objectives, and study questions. This organization helps to direct initial learning and assess areas where review is needed. The reader can approach the three parts individually, use specific areas for review, or look up a particular topic for immediate use. The strength of the handbook is its accessibility of information geared to U.S. and Canadian community health practice.

We are grateful for the suggestions and constructive

comments of colleagues who responded enthusiastically to our ideas. We are also indebted to our students at the University of British Columbia, Vancouver, who used the handbook in its early form and gave us much positive feedback. Our typists, Tere Rostworowski and Betsy Lam, coped with penciled notes and produced miracles during our revisions.

*L. Claire Bennett*
*Sarah Searl*

# Contents

**I  Introductory Concepts in Communicable Disease Control  1**

  1  Health Protection Measures for Communities  3

  2  Immunology  16

  3  Principles of Immunization  43

**II  Control of Communicable Disease by Immunization  55**

  4  Professional Responsibilities in Immunization Programs  57

  5  Current Routine Immunizations  70

  6  Immunization for Special Needs  86

**III  Communicable Diseases Not Presently Immunizable  111**

  7  Chickenpox: The Varicella Zoster Infections  113

  8  Hepatitis  119

9   Infectious Mononucleosis   131

10   Parasitic Conditions and Infections   137

11   Salmonella   157

12   Sexually Transmitted Diseases   167

13   Skin Conditions and Infections   208

14   Streptococcal Infections   219

15   Tuberculosis   228

Answers to Study Questions   253

Index          258

# COMMUNICABLE DISEASE HANDBOOK

# PART I

## INTRODUCTORY CONCEPTS IN COMMUNICABLE DISEASE CONTROL

The control of communicable disease occurs on two main fronts: protection of the people and protection of the environment. Part I introduces ideas basic to understanding principles of protection in both areas. The initial chapters discuss epidemiology, legislative action taken by communities to provide safe and healthy places to live and work, the body's immune response system, and immunization rationale. Part I, therefore, groups information and concepts that are used throughout the manual, so review of material in these early chapters is encouraged as readers work with the handbook.

# 1

# Health Protection Measures for Communities

When you have successfully completed this chapter, you will be able to:

1. Define epidemiology.
2. List the factors that contribute to the occurrence of communicable diseases.
3. Interpret rates used in compiling vital statistics.
4. Describe interventions using the primary, secondary, and tertiary prevention models.
5. Identify health protection programs in your community.

## WHAT IS EPIDEMIOLOGY?

Disease prevention and protection in the population and the environment demand a different approach than that used in caring for a person with a clinical illness. The study of disease prevention and protection in large groups is called **epidemiology**. By definition, epidemiology is the study of disease distribution or occurrence in a population. It is concerned with the patterns of disease and the multiple factors causing the disease. For example, not everyone who is exposed to a particular communicable disease will contract the infection. This is explained by thinking of disease as a balance mechanism: the virulence of the invading organism or agent balanced, or offset by, the resistance of the host, or the person being exposed to infection. The virulence of the infection is beyond our control, but resistance in the host is the result of factors such as age, sex, ethnicity, genetic background, nutritional status, occupational hazards, exposure to other pathogenic organisms, and the whole sociocultural and physical environment. Obviously, some of these factors are amenable to change, and this forms part of the work of epidemiologists. Intervening to improve or raise host resistance is a prime function of health care personnel, who draw implications for their work from knowing how epidemiologists approach the task of assessing disease patterns.

## Epidemiological Measurements

Epidemiologists study large populations and identify groups who are at highest risk of disease by reason of any or all of the preceding factors. Such large-scale studies yield data that are invaluable in analyzing the association of disease occurrence with population characteristics. In other words, in looking for patterns of disease occurrence, epidemiologists are alert to any correlation between certain disease and the presence of particular risk factors.

Epidemiologists measure the amount of disease in a population or community by relating established cases to a

population base. These measurements are stated as *rates*.
For example:

$$\text{Incidence rate} = \frac{\text{Number of cases in a time period}}{\text{Population in the same area in the same time period}}$$

Rates expressed in this manner represent a significant difference between clinical studies and epidemiological studies. **Clinical studies** concern the number of cases, or the numerator only (e.g., "A Study of 1,000 Cases of Gonorrhea"). **Epidemiological studies**, however, are concerned with presenting the number of people affected, or the *incidence*. of a disease, for a defined population base. The incidence is then expressed as a rate with numerator and denominator (e.g., "A Study of 1,000 Cases of Gonorrhea in a College Population of 23,000 Students").

Epidemiologists are further concerned with measuring the pattern of human life events, or the "hatch, match, and dispatch"! Measurements gained from compiling births, marriages, and deaths are called **vital statistics**; some typical rates are given in Table 1.1.

## Levels of Prevention

The present health care system is more effective in preventing certain diseases than others. This has given rise among health professionals to a term called **levels of prevention**, of which there are currently three.

*Primary prevention* ideally stops disease before it occurs. Fortunately, there is primary prevention in many instances; some examples are immunizations, pure food and

**Table 1.1** Birth, Mortality, and Morbidity Rates

Crude birth rate

$$\frac{\text{Number of registered births in a year}}{\text{Total population as of July 1}^b} \times 1{,}000^a$$

Crude death rate

$$\frac{\text{Number of deaths registered in a year}}{\text{Total population as of July 1}} \times 1{,}000$$

Maternal mortality rate

$$\frac{\text{Maternal deaths from all puerperal causes in a year}}{\text{Total number live births in same year}} \times 1{,}000$$

Infant mortality rate

$$\frac{\text{Number of deaths under one year in a year}}{\text{Total number live births in a year}} \times 1{,}000$$

Incidence rate

$$\frac{\text{Number of new cases within a given period of time}}{\text{Population at risk at beginning of that period}} \times 1{,}000$$

Prevalence rate

$$\frac{\text{Total number of cases of specific disease at a point in time}}{\text{Population at that point in time}} \times 1{,}000$$

[a] Number per 1,000 used to express proportion in these examples.

[b] Population at midpoint in time used if denominator size is changing.

water legislation, housing codes and standards, and health education. Primary prevention involves scrutiny and manipulation of the risk factors for disease at an individual, community, or population level.

It is in the arena of primary prevention that epidemiologists and the related health care services have much to share. It is apparent that with the escalating costs of acute care, future health care delivery will have to refocus its priorities onto primary prevention. Much is known about disease processes, yet a credibility gap remains between knowledge and action in relation to improved health. The classic example is cigarette smoking. Enormous amounts of data have been accumulated that relate smoking to deleterious effects on health, but it took nearly 20 years of sharing that information with the public to produce a significant change in U.S. and Canadian smoking habits. There has been vast improvement in the quality of our environmental health, but the future will bring greater emphasis on promoting a quality of life-style through primary preventive actions.

*Secondary prevention* is aimed at detecting disease early in the invasive process so that prompt and thorough treatment may begin. This early intervention may produce a cure, prevent disability, slow the progression of the disease, or return infective people to a noncommunicable state. Secondary prevention measures include screening programs such as those for glaucoma, cancer of the cervix, tuberculosis, and hearing loss. Screening programs are followed by thoroughly checking on the people screened out as at risk for the disease, with repeated follow-ups at future intervals as indicated. Another example of secondary prevention is prompt and thorough treatment in instances of cancer or tuberculosis to prevent further progression and yield a possible remission. Secondary prevention also includes the tracing and follow-up of contacts of known cases of infectious diseases such as gonorrhea or typhoid. When tracing is conscientiously done, the contacts will benefit from primary prevention!

*Tertiary prevention* is directed at restoring a person to the highest possible level of functioning after disease has left residual damage. Modern tertiary measures include the range of physical, social, and emotional rehabilitation resources that are available such as physiotherapy, occupational retraining and counseling, and financial services. Tertiary prevention implies close and frequent collaboration between the patient and the many support agencies often involved. This level of prevention also highlights ethical issues; clear communication between the patient and health worker is vital. For tertiary prevention to be meaningful, the first issue to be agreed on is the final goal of the support and intervention. The patient must be the one who articulates this and is then aided by skilled help; if not, the intervention becomes futile. Present-day rehabilitation has much to offer, but it requires effective management so that its diversity be harnessed for the good of the patient.

## COMMUNITY RESPONSE

The community health worker's client may be an individual, a family, a neighborhood, or a community. Clients can be helped to identify risk factors and initiate interventions to prevent disease; if this is not possible, the chance of serious side effects can be lessened. Day-to-day practice in the community gives the health professional many opportunities to use and benefit from epidemiology; the study of communicable disease is only one facet. The work surrounding contagious disease, however, has provided landmark advances in reducing human suffering with immeasurable improvement in both the length and quality of life.

## Collecting Information

Community health agencies are also responsible for collecting information on the incidence of certain diseases that are termed reportable or notifiable. Some of the reportable disease are measles, hepatitis, tuberculosis, sexually transmitted diseases, poliomyelitis, rubella, and streptococcal infections. Although reporting of these diseases may not be as accurate as morbidity rates would be, such information does point out trends. It is possible to plan and implement actions, based on weekly reporting, if there is a marked upswing in incidence. Monthly and annual reports usually seem to be dry reading, but we can see the impact of our work and plan future programs based on the patterns emerging from disease reporting. Communicable diseases often demonstrate seasonal fluctuations in incidence and cyclical variation in severity. For example, streptococcal infections and rheumatic fever have a higher incidence in the winter and spring; other communicable disease can be particularly severe in a given year after a mild form of infection has been experienced in prior years. Accurate diagnosis and meticulous reporting of notifiable disease enhances the community health worker's ability to be "forewarned and forearmed" in meeting the health needs of the community.

## LEGISLATIVE ACTION

Legislative action is taken by communities to protect citizens in many ways. Tax-supported programs are carried out by health agencies and reflect the philosophy of primary prevention. Typical programs include

1. *Protection of the water supply.* Regulations here include laws governing the digging of wells, chlorination and fluoridation, restricted access to watershed areas, and ongoing purity testing.

2. *Protection of the food supply.* Contaminated food can spread many of the same diseases as water, so there is close supervision of food sources, storage facilities, preparation, and serving. Legislation usually covers areas such as inspection of dairy herds and meat and poultry processing plants; maintenance of sanitary conditions in restaurants, including health status regulations for food handlers, and garbage disposal.

3. *Isolation and quarantine.* Depending on the communicable disease, regulations state how long an infected person and his or her contacts must be isolated from others. These regulations also protect communities against infectious diseases not indigenous to that area from being imported by travelers.

4. *Case finding and treatment.* An important aspect of disease control, case finding involves searching out and following up with treatment contacts of disease such as tuberculosis, salmonella, and gonorrhea.

5. *Sewage disposal and treatment.* Legislation governing the discharge of sewage is closely allied with protection of food and water supplies. Communities vary in

their treatment of sewage from holding ponds, aeration, percolation, disinfection, or a combination thereof. Local legislation also determines the point at which the treated sewage may be discharged.

6. *Supervision of public swimming pools and bathing beaches.* Since water provides an excellent transport medium for disease organisms, swimmers must also be protected. Public pools and beaches are regularly checked for their coliform count, since the coliforms are a fecal contaminant. Disinfectant chemicals in pools can be adjusted to lower the count, but beaches may be closed if the water is too contaminated for swimming.

7. *Established construction standards for private and public buildings.* Federal and local legislation is directed at making buildings safe. Regulations, or building codes, are more stringent for public buildings such as schools or churches, which are used by large groups; regulations apply to things such as exits, ramps and toilets accessible by wheelchairs, and fireproof or fire-retardant materials. Private and public buildings must provide a certain level of light, ceiling heights, quality of electricity, and the like.

Communities may enact additional bylaws to deal directly with a local or area concern. An example of this would be the setting up of a local clinic to cope with the health needs of a particular group of people, transient or resident. These local area needs may result from a temporary crisis, such as an influx of immigration, and will disband after the need disappears. Sometimes, however, a local response "fills a long-felt need" and becomes a permanent fixture in the community, such as a drop-in center for street youth. This situation will often stir a neighborhood into action to press governments for longer-term funding to keep a needed facility alive.

The various levels of government (federal, provincial or state, and municipal) share the responsibility for employing personnel to carry out these programs. Budgets are determined on a cost-sharing basis, with all levels cooperating in the program planning to avoid duplication of services.

## STUDY QUESTIONS

1. Four host factors that can contribute to the occurrence of disease are _____ , _____ , _____ , and _____ .

2. As a quantitative science, epidemiology measures and describes _____ of persons.

3. $\dfrac{\text{Number of persons developing a disease}}{\text{Total number at risk}}$ per unit of time expresses the _____ rate.

4. $\dfrac{\text{Number of persons with a disease}}{\text{Total number in that population}}$ at a particular time expresses the _____ rate.

5. Two examples of primary prevention are _____ and _____ .

6. Contact tracing and screening are two examples of _____ prevention.

7. A key concept in understanding tertiary prevention is _____ .

8. Case finding involves identification of and follow-up of _____ .

9. The exclusion from school of a child with a contagious condition is called _____ .

10. An official report notifying the local health authority of a disease is mandatory in certain communicable conditions such as _____ .

## BIBLIOGRAPHY

Archer, S. E., and R. P. Fleshman. *Community Health Nursing Patterns and Practice*, 2nd ed. North Scituate, Mass.: Duxbury Press, 1979. Ch. 9.

Benenson, A. S., Ed. *Control of Communicable Diseases in Man*, 12th ed. Washington, D.C.: The American Public Health Association, 1975.

Breslow, L. "Cigarette Smoking and Health." *Public Health Reports*, **95**(5), 451–455 (1980).

Friedman, G. *Primer of Epidemiology*, 2nd ed. New York: McGraw-Hill, 1980.

Fromer, M. J. *Community Health Care and the Nursing Process*. St. Louis: C. V. Mosby, 1979. Pp 56–232.

Fruchter, R. C., J. Boyce, and M. Hunt. "Missed Opportunities for Early Diagnosis of Cancer of the Cervix." *American Journal of Public Health*, **70**(4), 418–420 (1980).

Graham, S. "The Sociological Approach to Epidemiology." *American Journal of Public Health*, **64**(11), 1046–1049 (1974).

Henderson, D. A. "Smallpox Eradication." *Public Health Reports*, **95**(5), 422–426 (1980).

Hilbert, M. S. "Prevention." *American Journal of Public Health*, **67**(4), 353–356 (1977).

Kramer, B. M. "Behavioral Change and Public Attitudes Toward Public Health." *American Journal of Public Health*, **67**(10), 911–913 (1977).

LaLonde, M. *A New Perspective on the Health of Canadians*. Ottawa: Government of Canada, 1974.

Langmuir, A. D. "The Epidemic Intelligence Service of the Center for Disease Control." *Public Health Reports*, **95**(5), 470–477 (1980).

Leavell, H. R., and R. G. Clark. *Preventive Medicine for the Doctor in His Community: An Epidemiologic Approach*, 3rd ed. New York: McGraw-Hill, 1965. Pp. 19–28.

Lilienfeld, A. M. "Advances in Quantitative Methods in Epidemiology." *Public Health Reports*, **95**(5), 462–470 (1980).

Louria, D. B., A. P. Kidwell, M. A. Lanehar, et al. "Primary and Secondary Prevention Among Adults: An Analysis with Comments on Screening and Health Education." *Preventive Medicine*, **5**(4), 549–572 (1976).

MacFarlane, A. "The Derivation and Uses of Perinatal and Neonatal Mortality Rates." *The Journal of Pediatrics*, **98**(1), 61–62 (1981).

Marier, R. "The Reporting of Communicable Diseases." *American Journal of Epidemiology*, **105**(2), 587–590 (1977).

Mausner, J., and A. Bahn. *Epidemiology*. Philadelphia: Saunders, 1974.

Miller, C. A. "Issues of Health Policy: Local Government and the Public's Health." *American Journal of Public Health*, **65**(12), 1330–1335 (1975).

Miller, C. A., E. F. Brooks, G. H. De Friese, et al. "A Survey of Local Public Health Departments and Their Directors." *American Journal of Public Health*, **67**(10), 931–939 (1977).

Miller, C. A., B. Gilbert, D. G. Warren, et al. "Statutory Authorizations for the Work of Local Health Departments." *American Journal of Public Health*, **67**(10), 940–945 (1977).

National League for Nursing. *Statistical Reporting in Home and Community Health Services*. New York: National League for Nursing, 1977.

Navarro, V. "From Public Health to Health of the Public." *American Journal of Public Health*, **64**(6), 538–542 (1974).

Patterson, J. E. "Assessing the Quality of Vital Statistics." *American Journal of Public Health*, **70**(9), 944–945 (1980).

Rosenstock, I. M. "Prevention of Illness and Maintenance of Health." In J. Kosa, A. Antonovsky, and I. Zola, Eds., *Poverty and Health, a Sociological Analysis*. Boston: Harvard University Press, 1969. Pp. 168–190.

Sackett, D. L. "Screening for Early Detection of Disease: To What Purpose?" *Bulletin of the New York Academy of Medicine*, **51**(1), 39–52 (1975).

Terris, M. "The Epidemiologic Revolution, National Health Insurance and the Role of Health Departments." *American Journal of Public Health* **66**(12), 1155–1164 (1976).

# 2

# Immunology

When you have successfully completed this chapter, you will be able to:

1. Know the function of reticuloendothelial cells and the process of inflammation in combating infection.
2. List the factors involved in innate immunity.
3. Describe the two basic systems for adaptive immunity.
4. Explain the process of vaccination.
5. Recognize the allergic response.

*This chapter traces the role of the reticuloendothelial system (RES), which, along with the white blood cells, has a major protective function in humans. Included is a discussion of how the RES determines body response to antibody inoculation and a description of the allergic reaction. Guyton's*

This chapter is taken from FUNCTION OF THE HUMAN BODY, Fourth Edition, by Arthur C. Guyton. Copyright © 1974 by W.B. Saunders Company, Copyright © 1959, 1964, 1969, by W.B. Saunders Company, Reprinted by permission by Holt, Rinehart and Winston.

*text is a standard in its field, and its treatment of this important and complex system is thorough, clear, and concise.*

# THE RETICULOENDOTHELIAL CELLS

Reticuloendothelial cells are closely allied to white blood cells. They are primitive cells that have intense ability to phagocytize particles foreign to the body. However, in contrast to white blood cells, reticuloendothelial cells are mainly sessile, usually lining vascular and lymphatic channels. One of the most distinctive types of reticuloendothelial cells is the **Kupffer cells** that line the liver sinusoids, but similar cells line sinusoids of the spleen, the lymph nodes, and the bone marrow.

One will note that the reticuloendothelial cells are propitiously located for removal of invading organisms or toxins before they spread widely. For instance, large numbers of colon bacilli are absorbed from the large intestine into the portal blood, but almost none of these succeeds in passing through the liver sinusoids without being phagocytized by the Kupffer cells. Indeed, motion pictures have shown that a colon bacillus, on coming in contact with the membrane of a Kupffer cell, enters the cell within the next 1/100 of a second, illustrating the extreme propensity of these cells for removing foreign debris from the circulation.

The reticulum cells in the lymph nodes also play a special role in cleansing the body fluids, for all lymph must pass through the sinuses of lymph nodes before entering the blood. Therefore, fluids draining from an infected area, carrying with them live bacteria, are first cleansed by the lymph nodes prior to reaching the general circulation.

In virtually all tissues of the body are cells called **macrophages or tissue histiocytes** that have phagocytic properties almost identical with those of the reticulum cells in the lymph nodes and the Kupffer cells in the liver sinuses. The tissue histiocytes are also closely related to monocytes. Therefore, it is evident that the reticuloendothelial cells and white blood cells are all part of a single large system to cleanse the blood and tissues of bacteria, dead tissue debris, and other particulate matter.

## INFLAMMATION AND WALLING OFF OF INFECTED TISSUE AREAS

Another important process of preventing spread of infection is the process of inflammation which occurs in any tissue that becomes damaged. This process may be described as follows:

Damage to the tissues causes several substances to be released from the cells. One of these is **leukotaxine** and another is **histamine**. Leukotaxine is a complex of substances that attracts polymorphonuclear neutrophils from the blood stream into the infected area. Histamine, as well as some of the other products from the damaged tissues, increases the permeability of the capillaries in the inflamed tissues, which allows fluid, proteins, and white blood cells to leak almost unabated into the area. Then still other substances released by the damaged tissues activate the fibrinogen in the leaked fluid, and thereby cause the fluid to clot in the same manner that blood clots. Clotting of these fluids prevents their flow from the damaged tissue area into the surrounding areas and, therefore, provides so-called "walling off" of the inflamed tissue from the surrounding tissues. This is especially important if the damage to the tissues is caused by bacteria, because it prevents the spread of bacteria.

Once the infected or damaged area had been walled off, the neutrophils and monocytes rapidly destroy the bacteria or other invading agents; then comes clean-up of the debris by the macrophages (monocytes). One of the processes used by the macrophages to remove dead tissue is simply to digest the tissue: the lysosomes of the macrophages release their digestive enzymes which in turn digest many or most of the dead tissue in the walled-off area. The end-products that are formed, combined with the dead neutrophils and monocytes, make up the substance called pus.

Soon thereafter, the pus is either emptied to the exterior through a rupture in the skin, or it is absorbed. And finally, the processes of tissue repair begin, caused mainly be ingrowth of fibroblasts that generate new connective tissue. Most of the fibroblasts originate from other fibroblasts in the surrounding tissue, but some of them develop de novo from large lymphocytes.

## IMMUNITY

### Innate Immunity

One's ability to ward off disease is called immunity. The human body has a basic ability to resist almost all types of organisms or toxins that tend to damage the body. Much of this resistance is based on general functions of the body rather than some processes directed at specific disease organisms. This is called **innate immunity**. It includes such factors as the following:

1. Destruction of bacteria and organisms that are swallowed into the stomach by the acid secretions of the stomach and by the digestive enzymes.

2. Resistance of the skin to invasion by organisms.

3. Destruction of organisms or toxins by the white blood cells and the reticuloendothelial system.

4. Presence in the blood of certain chemical compounds which will attach to foreign organisms or toxins and destroy them. Some of the naturally occurring coagulants in the blood probably have this ability. However, one specific agent recently discovered is the substance interferon. This substance is formed by many of the body's cells when they become infected with viruses. It in turn is released into the circulating blood where it then attacks other virus particles before they invade additional cells. Thus, the presence of interferon in the circulating blood is probably of great importance in preventing devastating effects of viral diseases.

## Adaptive Immunity

In contrast to innate immunity, the body has a highly developed specialized system that allows it to develop specific immunity, called **adaptive immunity**, to specific invading organisms or toxins. In this system, the body is not naturally immune to the invading organism, and the body does not resist the invasion upon first exposure to the invader. However, within a few days to a few weeks after exposure, this special immune system will have developed extremely powerful resistance to the invader. Furthermore, the resistance will be highly specific for that particular invader and not for others. It is for this reason that this type of immunity is called "adaptive" immunity.

Adaptive immunity can bestow extreme protection against a specific invader. For instance, certain toxins, such as the paralytic toxin of botulism or the tetanizing toxin of tetanus can be protected against in doses as high as 100,000 times the amount that would, without immunity, be lethal. This is the reason why the process known as "vaccination" is so extremely important in protecting human beings against disease and against toxins, as will be explained in the course of this chapter.

### ANTIGENS

Since adaptive immunity does not occur until after first invasion by a foreign organism or toxin, it is clear that the body must have some mechanism for recognizing the initial invasion. Each toxin or each type of organism contains a specific chemical compound or compounds in its makeup that are different from all other compounds. In general, these are proteins, large polysaccharides, or large lipoprotein complexes, and it is they that cause adaptive immunity. These substances are called **antigens**.

### ROLE OF THE LYMPHOCYTES AND LYMPH NODES IN ADAPTIVE IMMUNITY

Located both in the lymph nodes and in special lymphoid tissue such as that of the spleen and of the submucosal areas of the gastrointestinal tract are special types of lymphocytes that react to invading antigens to elicit the adaptive immunity process. The lymphoid tissue is located in the body very advantageously to intercept the invading organisms or toxins before they can be spread too widely. For instance, the lymphoid tissue of the gastrointestinal tract is exposed immediately to any antigens invading through the gut. Likewise, the lymphoid tissue in the lymph nodes is exposed to antigens that invade from any of the peripheral tissues of the body. And, finally, the lymphoid tissue of the throat and pharynx (the tonsils and adenoids) is extremely well located to intercept antigens that enter by way of the respiratory tract.

## TWO BASIC SYSTEMS FOR ADAPTIVE IMMUNITY: HUMORAL IMMUNITY AND CELLULAR IMMUNITY

When lymphoid tissue is exposed to antigens it produces two different agents that in turn protect against the invading antigens. These are: (1) special protein molecules called **antibodies** that can react with the antigens to destroy either the antigens themselves or the host organisms, and (2) **sensitized lymphocytes** which also can attack and destroy either the antigen or its host.

The antibodies are released into the body fluids, and they circulate freely in the blood, also passing into the tissue spaces. Therefore, the immunity that is conferred upon the body by the antibodies is called **humoral immunity**.

The sensitized lymphocytes also circulate in the blood, but since lymphocytes are themselves living cells, the sensitized lymphocyte type of immunity is called **cellular immunity** or sometimes **lymphocytic immunity**.

*Formation of antibodies and sensitized lymphocytes in the lymph nodes.* Figure 2.1 illustrates the overall mechanism of

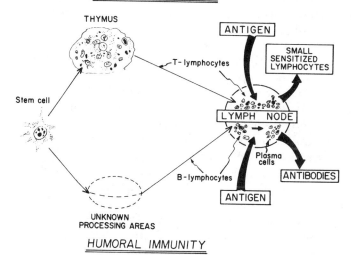

**Figure 2.1**  Formation of antibodies and sensitized lymphocytes by a lymph node in response to antigens. This figure also shows derivation of thymic and bursal lymphocytes responsible for the cellular and humoral immune processes of the lymph nodes.

adaptive immunity, showing to the right and below the formation of antibodies by the lymph nodes in response to antigens, and showing to the right and above the formation of sensitized lymphocytes. The basic mechanism by which the lymph nodes and other lymphoid tissue form the antibodies and sensitized lymphocytes is still unknown. However, we do know some of the basic cellular reactions that take place during the formation.

Upon entering the lymph node, the antigens become exposed to lymphocytes that are entrapped in the trabecular mesh of the nodes. In some way not presently known the antigen reacts with the lymphocytes and alters their protein producing abilities. Thereafter, these lymphocytes are capable of producing highly specific proteins which can directly attack the antigens. In the case of the humoral immunity system, these proteins are released as antibodies directly into the lymph, which then flows into the circulating blood to be spread throughout the body. In the case of the sensitized lymphocytes, the proteins remain in the lymphocytes, and the whole lymphocytes are released into the lymph and thence spread throughout the body.

The specific adaptive reactions that occur in the lymphocytes to cause production of antibodies and sensitized lymphocytes are, of course, the basis of the entire adaptive immunity system. Once a lymphocyte has been exposed to the antigen and has become adapted to form a specific type of immune protein, it thereafter will form that same specific type of protein for the remainder of its life. Therefore, this lymphocyte is said to be committed. And, after a lymphocyte has become committed, the original antigen is no longer needed—that is, the lymphocyte will continue producing the immune protein for months and sometimes even years after the antigen itself has been removed from the body.

## HUMORAL IMMUNITY

*Function of plasma cells.*   In the humoral immunity system, the committed lymphocytes divide many fold while still in the lymph nodes, and most of them are converted into **plasma cells**. The plasma cells in turn have an innate capacity for synthesizing especially large quantities of specific antibodies. In turn, the plasma cells dissolute and thereby dump their dissolved antibodies directly into the lymph that flows through the lymph nodes.

Once the antigen has disappeared from the lymph node, the remaining committed lymphocytes decrease their rate of division over a period of weeks. However, some of the committed lymphocytes nevertheless remain present in the lymph nodes for years, and subsequent exposure to the same type of antigen that caused the original commitment will elicit once again extremely rapid production of the same specific antibodies.

*Basic properties of antibodies and their function.* The antibodies are globulins, which are proteins of intermediate size. They circulate in the plasma of the blood and also diffuse in reasonable quantities through the pores of the capillaries into the tissue fluids.

Most antibodies develop two reactive sites which can react specifically with the antigen. This is illustrated in Figure 2.2, showing the antigen with any number of reactive sites but the antibodies with only two sites. The chemical reactive points in each reactive site of the antibodies are com-

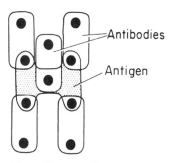

**Figure 2.2** Neutralization of an antigen by antibodies.

plementary to the chemical reactive points of each site of the antigen. That is, their physical arrangement, their number, and their chemical reactivities are such that they can combine with the complementary chemical reactive points on the specific antigens. Yet it would be very unlikely to find any other chemical compound with exactly the same combination of reactive points. It is for this reason that the antibodies are highly specific for specific antigens.

*Neutralization of antigens and precipitation.*    Some antigens that are very dangerous to the body are chemical substances, such as tetanus toxin, botulinum toxin, and toxins of other bacteria. The antibodies in general block the toxic effects of these substances by directly reacting with the antigens. Thus, as illustrated in Figure 2.2, the presence of large numbers of antibodies attached to a toxic antigen can destroy its toxic state. However, at times the presence of the antibodies does not completely block the toxicity. Yet, on the other hand, the antibodies can make the substance more susceptible to phagocytosis by white cells and reticuloendothelial cells, whereupon the digestive enzymes of these cells will eventually destroy the toxin.

The bivalent nature of the antibodies can also cause linkages between large numbers of antigen molecules, one of the valences of an antibody connecting with one antigen and the other valence connecting with the next antigen. When large numbers of antigens are linked in this way, the total complex becomes insoluble and will actually precipitate from the solution. Such precipitates are also highly susceptible to phagocytosis and destruction in the phagocytes.

*Destruction of cellular invaders by antibodies: Role of the "complement complex."*    When the invading agent is a cellular organism such as bacterium, a fungus, or even a cancer cell,

ANTIBODIES

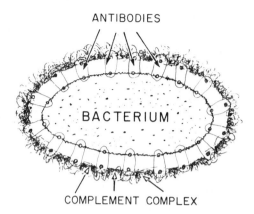

BACTERIUM

COMPLEMENT COMPLEX

**Figure 2.3**  Attachment of antibodies to a bacterium and envelopment of the bacterium by complement complex.

antibodies can often destroy the whole cellular organism. The process begins with attachment of antibodies to antigens in the membrane of the invading organism. This process is illustrated for a bacterium in Figure 2.3. However, attachment of the antibodies to the bacterium generally does not have a significant effect by itself to destroy the bacterium. Instead, the antibodies must in turn react with a series of protein substances in the circulating fluid called the complement complex before the bacterium can be destroyed.

The complement complex is a system of eleven different proteins. One of these proteins combines with the specific antibody that has already become attached to the bacterium, and then the other ten proteins of the complement complex combine successively with the first of these proteins. During the successive stages for combining additional complement proteins, the complement system acts as an **amplifying mechanism** because the first complement protein that combines with the specific antibody can eventually attract literally thousands of the additional complement proteins into the complex until the entire bacterium becomes totally engulfed by the complement system, even though the whole process has been initiated by only a few original specific antibodies attached to the bacterial cellular membrane.

Specific ways in which the combination of specific antibodies and complement complex destroy bacteria and other invading organisms include the following.

*Opsonization and phagocytosis.* Presence of the complement complex on the bacterium makes the bacterium susceptible to phagocytosis by white blood cells. This process is called **opsonization.** Without a specific antibody or without the complement complex most bacteria are relatively resistant to phagocytosis.

*Agglutination of bacteria.* The presence of complement complex makes bacteria sticky so that they tend to clump or **agglutinate.** This process immobilizes the bacteria until they can be exortized.

*Lysis of bacteria.* Lysis of bacteria means destruction of the bacterial membrane and dissolution of the bacterium. The complement complex contains digestive enzymes that are capable of destroying the bacterial cell membrane. Therefore, when a sufficient amount of complement becomes attached to the bacterial wall, the bacterium dissolutes, and its contents become dispersed. The same effect can occur for most other invading organisms including cancer cells, but generally it is the small sensitized lymphocytes that perform the lysis effect for the larger organisms.

*Types of disease against which the humoral mechanism protects.* In general, the humoral mechanism protects mainly against the bacterial diseases such as pneumonia, streptococcal infection, staphylococcus infection, and so forth. These are the types of disease that can cause rapid death of a person if they become rampant. On the other hand, the sensitized lymphocyte mechanism is more effective for the slowly developing infectious processes.

## CELLULAR IMMUNITY

*Release of sensitized lymphocytes in response to antigens.* Referring again to Figure 2.1, one can see above and to the right the release of small sensitized lymphocytes in response to antigen. As is also true in the humoral system, the presence of antigen commits certain specific lymphocytes in the lymph node to become sensitized against the invading antigen. Thereafter, these lymphocytes produce immune proteins that are probably similar to or identical with antibodies and that remain in the lymphocytes and become mainly attached to the membranes of the lymphocytes. Instead of secreting antibodies into the lymph, the whole lymphocytes pass into the lymph and then into the circulatory system.

Once the original lymphocytes of the lymph nodes have become committed, they then form large numbers of daughter cells which in turn divide many fold and release thousands of the small sensitized lymphocytes into the circulating body fluids. Furthermore, even after the antigen is completely gone, many committed lymphocytes still remain in the lymph node and continue to form new sensitized lymphocytes that will circulate months or years thereafter throughout the body. Furthermore, new exposure to the antigen, as is also true of the humoral system, causes once again extremely rapid increase in release of sensitized lymphocytes.

*Destruction of invading organisms by sensitized lymphocytes.* When sensitized lymphocytes come in contact with an invading organism—such as a cancer cell, a cell of a transplanted heart, a fungus cell, or so forth—the first effect is attachment of the sensitized lymphocyte to the invader as illustrated in Figure 2.4. This attachment presumably occurs between the antigens of the invading cell and the spe-

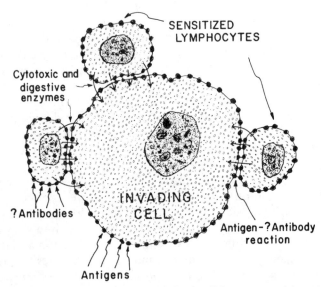

**Figure 2.4** Destruction of an invading cell by sensitized lymphocytes.

cific immune proteins in the membrane of the sensitized lymphocytes or, possibly, antibodies that are entrapped in the cell membrane. Attachment of the sensitized lymphocytes to the invading cell causes the lymphocytes to begin secreting cellutoxins and digestive enzymes that rapidly dissolve the membrane of the invading cell and digest the cell's contents. In the process, both the invading cell and the sensitized lymphocytes become destroyed, and their dissolved and digested products are absorbed into the body fluids.

*Types of organisms destroyed by sensitized lymphocytes.*    While the humoral-antibody mechanism for immunity is especially valuable against the acute bacterial diseases, the sensitized lymphocytes are a much more potent protective agent against the more slowly developing bacterial disease such as tuberculosis, brucellosis, and so forth. Also, sensitized lymphocytes are far more potent against cancer cells, cells of transplanted organs, and fungus organisms, all of which are far larger than bacteria. Finally, sensitized lymphocytes are especially potent against viruses, partially because viruses often do not cause potent antibodies and partly because sensitized lymphocytes can attack cells of the body that become infected by viruses, thus destroying both the cell and the infective agent together before the virus can multiply and spread too widely.

*Persistence of cellular immunity.*    Another feature of cellular immunity that is different from humoral immunity is its persistence. Humoral immunity usually lasts for a few months or a few years at most. On the other hand, once a person has developed intense cellular immunity against a foreign agent, this type of immunity usually lasts for many years, sometimes even for the entire lifetime of the person.

## Vaccination

The process of vaccination has been used for several centuries to cause adaptive immunity against specific diseases. A person can be vaccinated by injecting dead organisms which are no longer capable of causing disease but which still have their chemical antigens. This type of vaccination is used to protect against typhoid fever, whooping cough, and other types of bacterial diseases. Also, immunity can be achieved against toxins that have been treated with chemicals so that their toxic nature has been destroyed even though their antigens for causing immunity are still intact. This procedure is used in vaccinating against tetanus, botulism, and other similar toxic diseases. And, finally, a person can be vaccinated by infecting him with live organisms that have been **attenuated.** That is, these organisms have been grown either in special culture mediums or have been passed through a series of animals until they have mutated enough that they will not cause disease but will still carry the specific antigens. This procedure is used to protect against poliomyelitis, yellow fever, measles, smallpox, and many other viral diseases.

### THE PRIMARY AND SECONDARY RESPONSES

The initial response to vaccination usually does not begin for about seven days. Then, in the case of humoral immunity, the plasma concentration of antibody increases to a peak in about ten days to two weeks, but most of the antibodies disappear within six to eight weeks. This response is called the **primary response** to the vaccine; its time course is illustrated in Figure 2.5.

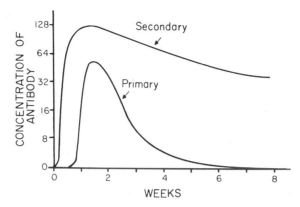

**Figure 2.5** Antibody responses to successive injections of vaccine.

When a subsequent injection of the same vaccine is given several weeks to several months later, a **secondary response** occurs, which is also illustrated in Figure 2.5. This time the release of antibodies begins within one to two days and reaches a peak in four to seven days. Furthermore, the antibody concentration becomes far greater and the antibodies last much longer. This explains why vaccination is usually performed by injecting an initial dose of antigen followed by one or more subsequent doses spaced weeks or months apart. It also explains why a **booster** dose of vaccine, sometimes given years later, can have high effectiveness in achieving a satisfactory degree of immunity against a specific organism.

## Active Versus Passive Immunity

Thus far, the adaptive immunity that we have discussed has all been **active immunity.** That is, the person's body develops either antibodies or sensitized lymphocytes in response to invasion of his body by a foreign antigen. However, it is possible to achieve temporary immunity in a person without injecting any antigen whatsoever into him. This is done by infusing either antibodies or sensitized lymphocytes or both into him from someone else or from some other animal that has been actively immunized against the antigen. The antibodies will last for two to three weeks, and during that time the person is protected against the invading disease. The sensitized lymphocytes will last for a few weeks if transfused from another person or a few hours to a few days if transfused from an animal. This transfusion of antibodies or lymphocytes to confer immunity is called **passive immunity.**

### TWO BASIC LYMPHOCYTE SYSTEMS FOR HUMORAL VERSUS CELLULAR IMMUNITY

The basic cause of the two different types of immunity, humoral and cellular, are two different types of lymphocytes in the lymph nodes. As shown in Figure 2.1, these two types of lymphocytes are called respectively **bursal lymphocytes** and **thymic lymphocytes,** or simply B-cells and T-cells. The origin of the thymic lymphocytes, which are responsible for cellular immunity, is the thymus gland, while the origin in the human being of the bursal lymphocytes responsible for humoral immunity is unknown. In birds the origin of these cells is an organ called the **bursa of Fabricius,** which accounts for the name. It is possible that some of the lymphoid tissue in the gastrointestinal tract is the source of these cells in the human being.

Both the thymic and the bursal lymphocytes come originally from primordial stem cells which are very similar to the original germinal epithelial cells from which the entire body is developed during embryonic life. The stem cells form primitive lymphocytes which lodge first in the thymus and bursa (of birds). In these organs the primitive lymphocytes are converted into special adaptive lymphocytes that are capable of subserving the functions of adaptive immunity. From the thymus and the bursa, the adaptive lymphocytes then migrate first into the blood and spread throughout the body; then they lodge in the lymph nodes and other lymphoid tissue such as the submucosal lymphoid tissue of the gut, the tonsils, and the spleen.

*Role of the thymus gland.*   One can understand that the thymus is an important organ for the process of cellular immunity. Most of the processing of lymphocytes by the thymus occurs shortly before birth of the baby and for a few months to a few years after birth. Therefore, beyond this period of time, removal of the thymus gland usually will not seriously impair the cellular immune process. However, removal several months before birth can completely prevent the cellular immunity mechanism. Since cellular immunity is the main type of immunity that causes rejection of transplanted organs—such as transplanted hearts, kidneys, and so forth—one can transplant organs almost with impunity if the thymus is removed from an animal a reasonable period of time before birth.

It is also believed that the thymus secretes a hormone that is capable of acting on the lymphocytes in the lymph nodes to increase their adaptive cellular immunity potential. It is especially believed that this hormone is needed during the early years of life to increase the activity of the cellular immunity process, though very little is yet known about either the nature or the function of this hormone.

## TOLERANCE OF THE ADAPTIVE IMMUNITY MECHANISM TO ONE'S OWN TISSUES

Obviously if a person should become immune to his own cells or other tissue elements, the immune mechanisms would destroy his own body. Fortunately, the immune mechanism normally recognizes the person's own tissues as being completely distinctive from those of invaders, and, for reasons not understood, the adaptive immunity system normally forms neither antibodies nor sensitized lymphocytes against the person's own antigens. This is known as **tolerance** to the body's own tissues.

Why tolerance occurs is almost completely unknown. However, it is known that when a body becomes swamped with tremendous quantities of antigens, the adaptive immune system sometimes becomes insensitive to these antigens. One of the theories for this is that such tremendous quantities of antigens reacting with committed lymphocytes causes destruction of those lymphocytes that become committed to these antigens. Therefore, no lymphocytes theoretically could become committed against the body's own tissues because of the tremendous swamping effect of the large quantities of antigens always acting on the thymus and lymph nodes.

*Autoimmune diseases.*    Unfortunately, the tolerance mechanism at times fails. When this occurs the immune system does then, unfortunately, form either antibodies or sensitized lymphocytes or both against the person's own tissues. This effect becomes more prevalent the older the person becomes. Therefore, many persons develop one or more diseases called autoimmune diseases that result from immunologic damage to specific tissues in the body. Some such diseases include rheumatic fever, in which the body has become immunized against tissues of the heart and joints; acute glomerulonephritis, in which the person has become immunized against tissues of the kidney to cause kidney disease; myasthenia gravis, in which immunity has developed against muscles throughout the body so that nerve impulses cannot be transmitted to the muscles, thus causing paralysis; and lupus erythematosus, in which the person becomes immunized against widespread numbers of tissues throughout his body, a disease that causes extensive immunologic damage, often enough to cause rapid death.

## ALLERGY

One of the unfortunate side effects of immunity is the development under some conditions of allergy. There are at least three different types of allergy, two of which occur under appropriate conditions in any person, and one of which occurs only in persons who have specific allergic tendency.

## Allergies That Occur in Normal People

### ANAPHYLAXIS

One type of allergy that can develop in a normal person is the phenomenon called anaphylaxis. This occurs only when the person is exposed suddenly to a large quantity of an antigen to which he is already strongly immunized. For instance, if a person has become strongly immunized to horse serum because he has been given serum previously to treat a disease, subsequent injection of horse serum into his circulating blood will occasionally cause such a severe anaphylactic reaction that it can actually kill him within a few minutes.

The mechanism of the severe reactions of anaphylaxis is the following: The large concentration of injected antigen reacts in the circulating blood and associated body fluids with large quantities of antibodies. When this reaction takes place in close association with white blood cells and with tissue cells, many of these cells in turn become highly permeable, and many actually dissolute, releasing large quantities of cellular substances into the fluids. Among these substances are histamine, serotonin, and even lysosomal digestive enzymes. The histamine itself can be very damaging. For instance, it causes dilation of peripheral blood vessels, with consequent fall of arterial pressure. It also causes the blood capillaries to become very leaky so that plasma leaks out of the circulation into the tissue fluids; and this too causes the arterial pressure to fall. It is usually the marked decrease in arterial pressure that is lethal. However, in addition, the histamine can cause bronchiolar spasm so that the person has difficulty breathing. Thus, one can understand that even the normal immune process when occurring extremely rapidly against large quantities of antigens can in itself be a lethal process.

## DELAYED REACTION ALLERGY

This type of allergy is caused by sensitized lymphocytes and not by antibodies. A typical example is a reaction to poison ivy. The toxin of poison ivy in itself does not cause much harm to the tissues. However, it does cause formation of sensitized lymphocytes. Then upon subsequent exposure to poison ivy toxin, the sensitized lymphocytes invade the tissues that have been exposed to the toxin and attack the local tissues where the toxin is present, thus often causing serious damage.

Similar reactions to that caused by poison ivy also result from certain drugs or chemicals that become exposed to the skin, particularly some cosmetics or household chemicals to which one's skin is often exposed.

## Allergy in the "Allergic" Person

Some persons have an "allergic" tendency. These persons have a propensity for forming an incomplete type of antibody called a **reagin** or a **sensitizing antibody.** These antibodies are very weak as antibodies and, therefore, cannot confer significant protection against the invading antigen. They also seem to become attached to cells throughout the body. When, upon subsequent exposure, a specific allergen (antigen) for the reagin enters the body, an allergen-reagin reaction takes place in close association with the attached cells, and damage to the cells occurs. This causes release of substances from the cells similar to those released during the anaphylaxis process—such as histamine, serotonin, and proteolytic enzymes. Therefore one can understand that different types of tissue damage can result.

Among the different types of allergies are:

*Hay fever.* In hay fever the allergen-reagin reaction occurs in the nose. Histamine released in response to this causes vascular dilation, with resultant increased capillary pressure and also increased permeability of the capillaries. As a result, fluid leaks into the tissues of the nose, and the nasal linings become swollen. Use of an antihistaminic drug can prevent this swelling reaction. However, additional products of the allergen-reagin reaction still cause irritation of the nose, still causing the typical sneezing syndrome despite drug therapy.

*Asthma.*   In asthma the allergen-reagin reaction occurs in the bronchioles of the lungs. Local products of this reaction cause direct stimulation of the smooth muscle of the bronchioles to cause resultant spasm. Consequently, the person has difficulty breathing until the reactive products of the allergic reaction have been removed. In asthma the cause of the smooth muscle contraction seems to be mainly other substances besides histamine because antihistaminics usually have only slight effect in ameliorating the symptoms of asthma.

*Urticaria.*   Urticaria is a condition in which swollen areas commonly called welts occur on the body in response to an allergic substance. This is generally caused by histamine released in local areas of the skin in response to an allergen penetrating the skin or in response to an allergen that enters the circulating body fluids. Here again, antihistaminics are of considerable value in treating the condition.

## STUDY QUESTIONS

1. Typical reticuloendothelial cells that line the liver sinusoids are called _____.
2. One of the processes used by the macrophages to remove dead tissue is _____.
3. The end products of this process combine with dead _____ and _____ to form pus.

4. The presence of _____ in the circulating blood attacks infections caused by viruses.

5. The chemical compound(s) that trigger the process of adaptive immunity are called _____.

6. The immunity that is conferred on the body by antibodies is called _____.

7. Antibodies are highly _____ for antigens.

8. Vaccination with "live" vaccines causes _____ immunity.

9. Plasma concentration of antibodies are higher and last longer in subsequent injections of a vaccine. This explains the effectiveness of _____.

10. _____ is a condition in which swollen areas commonly called welts occur on the skin in response to an allergic substance.

## BIBLIOGRAPHY

Gatti, R. A., O. Stutman, and R. A. Good. "The Lymphoid System." *Annual Review of Physiology,* **32,** 529–546 (1970).

Harboe, M. "Structure and Metabolism of Immunoglobulins. In E. E. Bittar and N. Bittar, Eds., *The Biological Basis of Medicine,* Vol. 4. New York: Academic Press, 1969. P. 197.

Heller, J. H. "Host Defence and the Reticulo-Endothelial System." In E. E. Bittar and N. Bittar, Eds., *The Biological Basis of Medicine,* Vol. 4. New York: Academic Press, 1969. P. 181.

Jandl, J. H. "The Spleen and Reticuloendothelial System." In W. A. Sodeman and W. A. Sodeman, Jr., Eds., *Pathologic Physiology,* 4th ed. Philadelphia: Saunders, 1967. P. 897.

Miescher, P. A., and H. J. Muller-Eberhard, Eds. *Textbook of Immunopathology,* Vols. I & II. New York: Grune & Stratton, 1968.

Miller, J. F. "The Thymus in Immunity." In E. E. Bittar and N. Bittar, Eds., *The Biological Basis of Medicine,* Vol. 4. New York: Academic Press, 1969. P. 225.

Potter, M. "Immunoglobulin-Producing Tumors and Myeloma Proteins of Mice." *Physiological Reviews,* **53**(3), 631–719 (1972).

Reite, O. B. "Comparative Physiology of Histamine." *Physiological Reviews,* **52**(3), 778–819 (1972).

Speirs, R. S. "How Cells Attack Antigens." *Scientific American,* **210**(2), 58–64 (1964).

Zmijewski, C. M. *Immunohematology.* New York: Appleton-Century-Crofts, 1968.

Zweifach, B. *The Inflammatory Process.* New York: Academic Press, 1965.

# 3

## Principles of Immunization

When you have successfully completed this chapter, you will be able to:

1. List important epidemiological methods used in the eradication and control of communicable disease.
2. Define herd immunity and explain its protective function in communities.
3. Recognize the personal and social forces that impact on immunization levels.
4. Describe the role of risk factors, placental passive immunity, and the immune response in developing vaccine administration schedules.
5. Devise health education objectives for immunization programs.

Protection with safe antigens against life-threatening communicable diseases is one of the basic tenets of public health. For centuries, health workers have struggled to reduce the awesome toll of lives claimed by the ravages of infectious diseases. The breakthroughs made by Jenner, Semmelweiss, Pasteur, and others irrevocably bettered the health of the world's populations. Effective vaccines against old killers have been developed within the lifetimes of many of our clients.

One of the most notable breakthroughs in disease control in recent years is smallpox. Closely monitored by the World Health Organization (WHO), the "pox" was narrowed down to a few pockets of infection, then virtually eradicated. It now appears that the WHO is safe in announcing that the smallpox threat is removed worldwide.

There is, however, a marked difference between **eradication** and **control** of an infectious disease. Smallpox eradication was possible because of the unique nature of that disease; for other contagious diseases, eradication may prove impossible. Control of contagion, or preventing an epidemic outbreak, uses the same epidemiologic methods as eradication, namely, case reporting (surveillance of the numbers with the disease) and primary prevention in the form of immunization and health teaching. These control methods will continue to shape health programs.

## IMMUNE LEVELS IN THE POPULATION

Case reporting and immunization programs work together: an effective innoculation program should obviously result in a lowered incidence of the particular disease under surveillance. For instance, since 1963 there have been more than 80 million doses of red measles vaccine given. The number of reported cases has gone from a pre-1963 total of about 500,000 to a total of about 35,000 in 1975

(Krugman, 1977). Because of their potential to infect large numbers of people rapidly, most infectious diseases are reportable and communities, therefore, can monitor the pattern of disease and plan their programs.

At the community level, public health agencies gather data on immunization levels in the population. For example, one northwestern Canadian city reported that 80% of the first-grade schoolchildren had sufficient protection against diptheria, polio, rubeola, rubella, and tetanus (Metropolitan Health Services of Greater Vancouver, Canada, 1978).

A value such as 80 out of 100 is often called **herd** immunity. The goal of immunization programs is to increase the percentage immunized and lower the numbers not protected. In other words, the members of the population ("herd") who are immunized exert a protective influence over those who are not, and this tends to keep potential epidemics under control. Significant and exciting conquests have given community health professionals effective weapons against disease. Ironically, this now presents a new battle front: complacency.

## HEALTH EDUCATION

There is an ongoing and urgent need to educate the public and professionals to counter this growing complacency, which is rooted in a variety of factors. From the professional viewpoint, many practicing doctors and nurses have never witnessed the onslaught of dreaded killers such as diptheria or poliomyelitis (Sampson, 1974). This out-of-sight, out-of-mind attitude carries over to the public, which, in turn, consists of younger parents who themselves have grown up with scant knowledge of the severity of these diseases. Theoretically, there are other infectious diseases, such as red measles that could also be eradicated if immunization levels were higher.

Studies have cited other factors contributing to complacency, such as more mobile families, immigrant families unfamiliar with U.S. and Canadian health programs, and inadequate knowledge of the efficacy of vaccines (Witte, 1975; Markland & Durand, 1976).

For health care workers in many outpatient settings, sufficient information on previous vaccinations is often unavailable due to the nature of the setting (e.g., prisons), the transient life-style of the individual or family, and the failure of responsible adults to keep accurate records of the immunizations they or their children have received (Witte, 1975).

The health care provider can audit immunization status records of people directly under their care. Instructing vaccinees of the importance of adequate record keeping can also insure that sufficient inoculations are carried out.

There is international agreement that immunizing children is a top priority, but disagreement exists as to the best method of achieving high "herd" levels in the under age 12 population. In Canada, there is agreement on a standardized national immunization schedule and an impetus to increase public awareness of immunization by educational methods (LeFort, 1979). The United States has made proof of immunization mandatory for children entering school (Anthony, 1977). In other countries, certain immunizations may be legally required, while others are optional, depending on the incidence of particular diseases. This difference in approach highlights one of the controversies surrounding mass immunization programs. Can individuals be required to prove that they are not disease risks to the community, or is such a requirement an infringement on personal rights? There are competent people arguing either side, and the debate continues (Braff, 1978).

Regardless of the method used to achieve better immune levels, families and clients must receive basic teaching about immunization in general and the vaccines in particular. Nurses and other community health workers can direct their energy toward lessening the negative impact of the other complacency factors. Organizing groups for immigrant parents with preschool children is one solution, with aspects of health in the new country, including immunizations, a topic for presentation and discussion. Ongoing health teaching by community health nurses in schools is another way of increasing knowledge about immunization. Lowered attendance in immunization programs can have serious repercussions for the individual, the family, and the health care system. The recurrence of some of these diseases, or the still high numbers of reported cases in others, means that our work as health care professionals in communicable disease is far from finished.

One of the problems facing community health workers is interpreting the constantly changing schedules and procedures to people in our care. Clients should be made aware that changes are due to ongoing studies being done on vaccines and the efficiency with which antibody response is promoted and maintained. An understanding of this principle will alert patients to inquire about the need of reinforcing doses or boosters.

# Vaccines and the Immune Antibody Response

Antibody response is based on three main factors: (1) the type of antigen used (live, killed, attenuated, adsorbed, etc.), (2) the ability of an antigen to stimulate antibody response (called the **antigenic quality** of the vaccine), and (3) the individual's response to the antigen (the antibody production by the reticuloendothelial system, or RES).

**Live vaccines** (e.g., rubella, yellow fever) usually give lasting immunity or immunity for many years. This means that the vaccine provokes an antibody titer that remains at a level high enough for protection. **Toxoids, killed, attenuated,** and **adsorbed** vaccines all need reinforcing doses at regular intervals to boost antibody response and keep it at a level high enough for protection. (If necessary, review the earlier discussion in Chapter 2).

## ADSORBED VACCINES

The standard fluid toxoid has shown excellent antigenic properties over the years. The drawbacks, however, are rapid absorption and elimination of the soluble toxoid by the body. This leads to a less than optimum antitoxin response that necessitates booster doses of relatively high dosage. Toxoids are improved by adding a substance such as aluminum salts. These cause the toxoid to precipitate and be held on the surface of the added substance. These substances are called **adjuvants**; in essence, they bond with the toxoid material. This bonding is called adsorption, and the resulting product is an adsorbed vaccine.

This improved adsorbed vaccine stimulates a higher antibody titer because the precipitate, or adjuvant, material remains at the injection site. It is released slowly over a more prolonged period of time. This is called the adjuvant, or depot, effect. Because the antibody titer is better, both the toxoid content and the dosage can be reduced.

## STUDYING RISKS:
## VACCINE VERSUS DISEASE

Another aspect of the ongoing study of immunological response is that of risk factors. The latter also account for changes in administration programs as more is learned. In other words, the risk of immunizing with a vaccine must be weighed against the positive effects of protection. The most recent example is smallpox. We no longer routinely vaccinate with smallpox, since the disease risk is virtually nonexistent (i.e., there is no need for protection) and the risks of inoculation sequelae are greater. These risks and possible sequelae make preimmunizing screening a must. Screening of the vaccinee is further discussed in Chapter 4.

*The immune antibody response in infants.*   Risk factors and immune response are especially pertinent when initial immunization is given to infants. Some antibodies are small enough to pass through the placenta and provide natural passive immunity in the fetus that lasts for varying lengths of time after delivery. Rubella and rubeola antibodies, received from the mother, may last up to the baby's first birthday and inactivate immunizing antigens. Therefore the recommended time for immunizing the child against rubella and rubeola to produce an active immunity is after the first birthday. Other antibodies, such as pertussis, do not cross the placenta, so the infant has no immunity from the mother and, therefore, needs to be immunized early.

Remember that for the infant to benefit from placental passive immunity, the mother must have an adequate antibody titer in her own bloodstream. This means that adults, not just children, must keep their inoculation boosters up to date.

The immaturity of the infant's immune system must also be considered. For example, at age 2 to 3 months, when injections of combined diphtheria, pertussis, and tetanus vaccine are usually started, the immune response is weak. For this reason, relatively large doses of antigen are given and repeated in a series of three or four doses to achieve maximum antibody production.

## COPING WITH CHANGE

The pioneer work in infectious disease control opened a floodgate of inquiry and knowledge. Protection of the individual and the environment has surpassed the wildest prophecies of 100 years ago yet, as more is learned about antibody response, more questions are raised and pursued. Immunology, or the study of vaccines and their effect in humans, proceeds apace on many fronts, including the search for new vaccines for old disease problems. Some of these new vaccines will be discussed in Parts II and III. It often seems that change in vaccine schedules and administrative practices comes all too often and is a source of anxious frustration to health workers involved in immunization programs as they strive to keep themselves and their clients up to date. Although the organizational routines change, the basic principles remain: safe vaccines given to a wide population base and accompanied by careful monitoring.

## STUDY QUESTIONS

1. Control of communicable diseases is accomplished by case reporting or _____.
2. Primary preventative control measures for communicable diseases include _____ and _____.
3. Potential epidemics are prevented in part by high percentages of persons immunized. This is called _____.
4. Low immunization rates in children reflect professional complacency due to _____.
5. Family complacency factors leading to failure to immunize are related to _____, _____, and _____.
6. The problem of low rates of immunization in the U.S. population has been addressed by _____.
7. In Canada, national _____ methods are being used to insure early, adequate immunizations.
8. Adsorbed vaccines stimulate a higher antibody titer due to the _____ or _____ effect.
9. Changes in vaccine administration program mainly result from study of _____ and the _____.
10. Recommended times for immunizing children against rubella, rubeola, and pertussis are based on the role of _____ immunity.

## BIBLIOGRAPHY

Anthony, N., M. Reed, A. M. Leff, et al. "Immunization: Public Health Programming Through Law Enforcement." *American Journal of Public Health,* **67**(8), 763–764 (1977).

Braff, E. H. "Rubella Vaccination: Society and the Individual." *The New England Journal of Medicine,* **299**(10), 556 (1978).

Connaught Laboratories. *A Compendium of Connaught Adsorbed Vaccine.* Ontario: Connaught Laboratories, 1980.

Constanzo, G. A. "Promoting Child Health: The Work of the Community Health Department and the International Year of the Child." *Canadian Journal of Public Health,* **70**(4), 240–242 (1979).

"General Recommendations on Immunization." *Morbidity and Mortality Weekly Report,* **29**(7), 76, 81–83 (1980).

Guyton, A. C. *Function of the Human Body,* 4th ed. Philadelphia: Saunders, 1974. Pp. 70–79.

Henderson, D. A. "Smallpox Eradication." *Public Health Reports,* **95**(5), 422–426 (1980).

Jensen, M. D., R. C. Benson, and I. M. Bobak. *Maternity Care.* St. Louis: Mosby, 1977. Pp. 201, 688.

Krugman, S. "Present Status of Measles and Rubella Immunization in the United States: A Medical Progress Report." *The Journal of Pediatrics,* **90**(1), 1–12 (1977).

Krugman, S. "Rubella Immunization: Progress, Problems and Potential Solutions." *American Journal of Public Health,* **69**(3), 217–219 (1979).

Le Fort, S. "Problem of Immunization in Canada." *The Canadian Nurse,* **75**(1), 26–30 (1979).

Markland, R. E., and D. Durand. "An Investigation of Socio-Psychological Factors Affecting Infant Immunizations." *American Journal of Public Health,* **66**(2), 168–170 (1976).

Medical News. "Gaps Remain in Vaccine Dike Against Many 'Common' Diseases." *Journal of the American Medical Association,* **233**(13), 1347–1348 (1975).

Metropolitan Health Service of Greater Vancouver. *Report of Immunization Status in Selected Grades: School District No. 39.* Vancouver, B.C.: Metropolitan Health Service, June 1978.

Robbins, K. B., D. Brandling-Bennett, and A. R. Hinman. "Low Measles Incidence: Association with Enforcement of School Immunization Laws." *American Journal of Public Health,* **71**(3), 270–274 (1981).

Sampson, P. "Immunization vs. Complacency: Are We Ready for the Challenge?" *Journal of the American Medical Association,* **229**(12), 1557–1570 (1974).

Schoenrich, E. "The Potential of Health Education in Health Services Delivery." *Public Health Reports,* **89**(1), 3–7 (1974).

Vernon, T. M., J. S. Conner, B. S. Shaw, et al. "An Evaluation of Three Techniques for Improving Immunization Levels in Elementary Schools." *American Journal of Public Health,* **66**(5), 457–460 (1976).

Wintermeyer, L., and M. G. Myers. "Measles in a Partially Immunized Community." *American Journal of Public Health,* **69**(9), 923–927 (1979).

Witte, J. J., and N. W. Axnick. "The Benefits from 10 Years of Measles Immunization in the United States." *Public Health Reports,* **90**(3), 205–207 (1975).

# PART II

## CONTROL OF COMMUNICABLE DISEASE BY IMMUNIZATION

Part I introduced ideas and knowledge basic to community health practice in disease control. Part II builds on these foundation concepts and applies them to immunization programs in the community. As the title implies, there is significant control of certain contagious diseases by the giving of antigens, or vaccines, against those diseases to large numbers of people. The etiology of the diseases covered in Part II is not included because the diseases are controlled; the focus in the following chapters is on the issues faced by nurses and allied health workers who are involved in carrying out immunization programs with the public.

# 4

## Professional Responsibilities in Immunization Programs

When you have successfully completed this chapter, you will be able to:

1. Screen vaccinees for general precautions or contraindications to immunization.
2. Discriminate between a general and local reaction to immunization.
3. Describe the anaphylactic reaction and emergency treatment protocols.
4. Carry out record-keeping responsibilities with clients.
5. Apply principles of asepsis and safe handling of antigens when administering biologicals.

Immunization programs are an example of primary preventive care. The responsibilities are considerable, since there are risks to the client in receiving any vaccine. The responsibilities and risks are dealt with in this chapter, under the topic headings of screening the vaccinee, emergency treatment of anaphylaxis, maintaining records for the client and the health agency, and the safe handling and administration of antigen products.

The concomitant responsibility to a well-managed program is the quality of the health teaching given to raise the client's level of health knowledge. Quality health teaching demands that the practitioner have a sound working knowledge of immunity, allergy, and risk factors and be able to apply that knowledge to the person receiving the vaccine, adult or child. (If necessary, review Chapter 3 for material on immune response and allergy.)

## SCREENING THE VACCINEE

Health teaching in immunization programs begins with a careful screening of the patient at every visit; this screening is not to be eliminated because of a previous history of trouble-free injections. In a short period of time, many factors can change a person's suitability for vaccination; this is especially so with children. The very act of taking time to validate information with a patient may in itself raise questions and answers not considered before and presents an opportunity for free exchange of new information. There are instances in which people should not be immunized, so a general screening is done first, followed by an interview to gain specific information about the person to be inoculated.

# General Precautions or Contraindications to Immunizing

There is no priority intended in the following list; each item is equally important.

- Children with a history of seizures (convulsions) after having pertussis (whooping cough) vaccine should never again receive that vaccine, either alone or in any combination of vaccine.
- People with a history of a convulsive disorder (epilepsy or the like) should be immunized by their private physician.
- No immunizations should be given to anyone with chronic kidney disease.
- Extreme care should be taken with people who have a history of allergies, especially to antibiotics such as penicillin and streptomycin.
- Live vaccines may suppress tuberculin sensitivity; therefore, the tuberculin (PPD or Mantoux) test should be done before immunizing or after a 30-day interval.

## Interviewing

Screening out the preceding contraindications is followed by a brief interview to ascertain the particular patient's current health status. Again, no priority is intended by the listing.

- Is the person to be inoculated well (i.e., no intercurrent infections being treated with medication)?

- Is the person taking any medications of any kind, especially steroids or antibiotics?
- Has the person recently been under a doctor's care?
- In the instance of a woman of childbearing age, is she pregnant? Pregnancy does not entirely rule out all inoculations, but it is certainly a specific contraindication to some, such as certain live vaccines.
- Did the person experience any reactions to previous injections? The **reaction** referred to here is not immediate or life-threatening anaphylaxis, but one that occurs hours later. It is much less severe but can cause considerable discomfort. Most people experience no difficulty with immunization, but this is an instance where such information may need reinforcing. In other words, clients may not report reactions because they erroneously thought discomfort was to be expected. Patients need to be reassured that with many vaccines there is no anticipated reaction. They also need an explanation of what is meant by the term reaction, what they can do to relieve the discomfort, and that it is essentially not serious but may require alteration in their immunization program. Lower-grade reactions that occur later may be general (systemic) or local. The latter produces inflammation, tenderness, and possible induration at the injection site for a few hours immediately afteward; the reaction is relieved by cold compresses and age-appropriate doses of acetylsalicylic acid (ASA) or Tylenol. The former produces chills, fever, sweating, general malaise and, infrequently, nausea and vomiting; it is best relieved by rest and ASA or Tylenol, if tolerated. In either instance, the reaction does not mean immunization must be abandoned, but

care must be taken with future injections. One technique is to administer the ASA or Tylenol promptly to forestall the discomfort.

The reaction may be mainly local or general, but it is often a combination of the two, since they are due to the direct irritating effect of the inoculated material. In both instances, the reaction does not usually last longer than 36 to 48 hours and is usually over in 12 to 24 hours.

In addition to the overall contraindications, precautions, and the individual interview, certain vaccinees need special attention and related client teaching. These specialized concerns are included in the discussion of the individual antigens in Chapters 5 and 6.

## EMERGENCY TREATMENT OF ANAPHYLAXIS

Occasionally, a person experiences an overwhelming allergic reaction to an antigen. (Refer also to previous discussion in Chapter 3.) This marked hypersensitivity may be a result of previous exposure to the antigen, but it can also occur without previous known antigen exposure in people with a history of eczema, urticaria, asthma, and hay fever. This profound reaction, called **anaphylaxis** or acute hypersensitivity, is a life-threatening emergency and is the prime reason for careful screening and for requesting that vaccinees wait a minimum of 20 minutes after an injection. Anaphylactic reactions are of three main types.

1. *Immediate anaphylaxis* occurs within minutes as a result of a marked antigen-antibody combination at the surface of the cells. Histamine is rapidly produced by the cells.

This acute histamine poisoning varies from person to person; the outcome is primarily cardiovascular or respiratory.

In the **cardiovascular reaction**, the patient experiences extensive vasodilation leading to a rapid drop in blood pressure accompanied by shock and loss of consciousness. The histamine produces a triple effect on the skin: pallor, followed by urticaria, and then welts plus a scarlet flushing.

During the **respiratory reaction**, the histamine poisoning causes bronchospasm leading to edema of the glottis with asthma, then cyanosis and asphyxia.

**A note to remember:** both the respiratory and cardiovascular reactions may be seen in combination in any person.

Treatment of immediate anaphylaxis uses epinephrine hydrochloride (adrenalin) 1:1,000 (0.1% solution) to counter the effect of the histamine poisoning. A typical treatment pattern is outlined below. It involves the immediate use of subcutaneous adrenalin coupled with emergency support (see Immunization Briefs in bibliography).

**Adrenalin Dosage:**

| Age | Weight (2.2 lb = 1 kg) | Recommended Dosage Epinephrine 1:1,000 |
|---|---|---|
| 3–12 months | 5–12 kg | 0.05–0.1 ml |
| 1–6 years | 12–23 kg | 0.1–0.2 ml |
| 6–12 years | 23–50 kg | 0.2–0.3 ml |
| 12 years and older | — | 0.3 ml |

**Emergency Support:**

- The recommended adrenalin dosage is given into the site of injection.

- Apply a tourniquet to the arm above the injection site **for no longer than 20 minutes.**
- In the opposite arm, give 0.05 ml per minute of 1/1,000 adrenalin up to a maximum of 0.2 ml.
- Maintain the airway and give oxygen if it is available.
- Get the patient to a hospital as quickly as possible, accompanied by a health professional and additional adrenalin.
- If a tourniquet is not used, the original dose of adrenalin may be repeated 15 minutes later.

2. *Encephalopathy* is another grave reaction occurring some hours after the injection. The cause is also a marked antigen-antibody combination, but the location now is the brain. The symptoms are convulsions and unconsciousness. Encephalopathy is also an emergency requiring immediate medical care. First-aid measures include lying the victim down and maintaining an airway.

3. *Delayed allergic reactions* are seen several days after an injection, usually from four to 10 days, and typically on the seventh or eighth day. Those symptoms include headache, fever, malaise, possible skin rash, lymphadenopathy, and arthralgia. Treatment is usually antihistamines and/or steroids or, occasionally, ephedrine or adrenalin.

The general principle underlying these descriptions is that the sooner the reaction is witnessed, the more severe and life threatening it is likely to be. Counsel patients to wait at least 20 minutes after receiving any antigen.

Health teaching is not intended to frighten patients; however, both the professional and the client must be aware of possible reactions and maintain a healthy respect for the properties of the vaccines used.

## MAINTAINING RECORDS

Concurrent with screening is the responsibility to give clients as much information about the vaccine as they need and want. In many instances, nurses have been guilty of using jargon names and initials for immunizations and have neglected to give vaccinees full and complete descriptions. Too many parents simply refer to the primary series in infancy as "baby shots." School-age children respond enthusiastically to preclinic teaching sessions designed to increase their knowledge of the immune process and "what they're getting in the arm."

Information sharing extends to records. Too often recipients of the vaccine are not given permanent records; they can hardly be taken to task for faulty recall! Private physicians keep their own office records, and parents are frequently at a loss to know what protection has been given their children. A full, up-to-date record is an entitlement. Community health agencies must also be meticulous in updating records, particularly when proof of immunization status is required for school entrance or overseas travel. The permanent record is also the logical place to note any reaction and the subsequent immunizing rationale.

## SAFE HANDLING OF ANTIGENS

**Antigens**, or biologicals, as they are sometimes called, require careful handling to prevent contamination and preserve their properties. This care includes

- Constant refrigeration but no freezing.
- Keeping antigens on ice packs when they must be out of the refrigerator and keeping this time as short as feasible.
- Observing expiration dates and replacing bottles in original boxes.
- Protection from exposure to sunlight.
- Cleansing rubber-topped bottles with disinfectant.
- Reading product information included in vaccine boxes, knowing possible vaccine abnormalities (such as clouding or lumping of the substance), and discarding any product that looks suspicious.

Some antigens require specific handling techniques that are outlined in the brochure in the product box. These brochures contain a wealth of information and are worth reviewing from time to time.

## Administration Procedure

Before giving any antigen, a syringe loaded with the appropriate dose of epinephrine should be readied and left in the administration area until all injections are completed and the last patient has waited a minimum of 20 minutes. The waiting period keeps vaccinees under observation for any possible immediate reaction.

Most antigens are currently given **subcutaneously**, using the deltoid muscle in the upper arm. The exceptions to this are oral polio, immune serum globulin (intramuscular), and smallpox (puncture or scratch).

This traditional, subcutaneous route is likely to change in the near future. Europe and some parts of the United States have used adsorbed vaccines for some time, and this use is increasing. **Adsorbed vaccines** are administered intramuscularly into the outer aspect of the midthigh or the deltoid. There is some disagreement as to which is the most appropriate site. The decision regarding the site of administration should be made after consultation with the vaccine manufacturer and local health and medical personnel. These vaccines have significant differences other than injection site and method and are discussed in greater detail in Chapter 3.

Both subcutaneous and intramuscular methods demand strict asepsis, efficient skin cleansing of the injection site with a suitable antiseptic, and rotation of injection sites when using adsorbed vaccines in the primary series.

The use of needles and syringes poses risks other than possible allergic reactions to patients. The possible sequelae of any immunization are a localized abscess at the injection site or syringe-transmitted hepatitis. A separate needle or disposable syringe must be used for each person.

## STUDY QUESTIONS

1. Children who have experienced _____ after receiving pertussis vaccine should never again receive that vaccine.
2. Chronic kidney disease is a _____ to any vaccine.

3. The tuberculin (PPD or Mantoux) test should be done before _____ or after a _____ day interval.

4. Pregnancy (does, does not) rule out all inoculations.

5. A technique for decreasing potential reactions to inoculations due to their irritating effect of the vaccine is to administer _____ promptly.

6. Anaphylaxis can occur when an antigen is injected into a person who is _____ to that antigen.

7. The substance released in this severe reaction to immunization is _____, which can cause bronchial spasm as well as lethal decreases in arterial pressure.

8. Preventing severe complications of acute allergic reactions includes _____, _____, and _____.

9. Adsorbed vaccines differ from traditional antigens in that they are administered _____ in the outer aspect of the _____ or the _____.

10. Two risks associated with the use of needles and syringes are _____ and _____.

## BIBLIOGRAPHY

Brown, M. S. "What You Should Know About Communicable Diseases and Their Immunizations." *Nursing 75*, **5**(9), 70–74 (1975).

Chow, M. P., B. A. Durrand, M. N. Feldman, et al. *Handbook of Pediatric Primary Care*. New York: Wiley, 1979. Pp. 48–49, 1955.

Connaught Laboratories. *A Compendium of Connaught Adsorbed Vaccines.* Ontario: Connaught Laboratories, 1980.

"General Recommendations on Immunization." *Morbidity and Mortality Weekly Report,* **29**(7), 76, 81–83, (1980).

Guyton, A. C. *Function of the Human Body,* 4th ed. Philadelphia: Saunders, 1976. Pp. 78–79, 140–151.

Harmon, A. L., and D. C. Harmon. "Anaphylaxis—Sudden Death Anytime." *Nursing 80,* **10**(10), 40–43 (1980).

Hingson, R. "Obtaining Optimal Attendance at Mass Immunization Programs." *Public Health Reports,* **89**(1), 53–64 (1974).

*Immunization Briefs.* British Columbia Ministry of Health. Victoria, B.C.: Province of British Columbia, 1981.

Jawetz, E., J. L. Melnick, and E. A. Adelberg. *Review of Medical Microbiology,* 12th ed. Los Altos, Calif.: Lange, 1976. Pp. 156–158.

Loebl, S., G. Spratto, E. Heckheimer, and A. Wit. *The Nurse's Drug Handbook,* New York: Wiley, 1977. Pp. 8, 448–449.

Modlin, J. F., K. Hermann, A. D. Branding-Bennett, et al. "Risk of Congenital Abnormality After Inadvertent Rubella Vaccination of Pregnant Women." *The New England Journal of Medicine,* **294**(18), 972–974 (1976).

Murphy, M. A. and M. S. Brown. "Health Maintenance for Children." In A. Reinhardt and M. Quinn, Eds., *Current Practice in Family-Centered Community Nursing.* St. Louis: Mosby, 1977. Pp. 206–208.

Quiring, J. D., and R. E. Rubeck. *Basic Nursing Skills: A Self-Instructional Approach.* North Scituate, Mass.: Duxbury Press, 1977.

Sampson, P. "Immunization vs. Complacency: Are We Ready for the Challenge?" *Journal of the American Medical Association,* **229**(12), 1557–1558, 1569, 1570 (1974).

Williams, J. "EPIDEMIC—What to do Before a Mass Immunization Program." *The Canadian Nurse,* **77**(7), 54–55 (1981).

Witte, J. J., and N. W. Axnick. "The Benefits from 10 Years of Measles Immunization in the United States." *Public Health Reports,* **90**(3), 205–207 (1975).

# 5

# Current Routine
Immunizations

When you have successfully completed this chapter, you will be able to:

1. Discuss basic immunizations with parents.
2. Describe an immunization schedule for infants and children.
3. Explain tests used to determine antibody titer and immune response and their use in clinical practice.
4. Recognize contraindications to current routine immunizations.
5. Prevent infectious diseases of infants and young children through adequate and safe immunization practices.

Inoculation programs afford primary prevention for many communicable diseases. This chapter discusses the immunizations routinely offered by most public health agencies to control diphtheria, mumps, pertussis (whooping cough), poliomyelitis, rubella (German measles), rubeola (red measles), and tetanus.

These antigens are called **basic** vaccines in community practice because they are fundamental to protection of the public's health. They are given routinely to infants and children as an initial or primary series of injections. Many health agencies supply these vaccines free or at low cost to the public and private physicians.

**Schedules** for giving vaccines are influenced by factors such as ongoing immunogenic study, local area needs and budgets, supply and demand of the vaccine, and knowledgeable personnel. With all these factors in operation, it is no surprise that schedules frequently change! For example, a health agency may decide its own local schedule in response to the amount of budget money available or to a concern in the area such as a measles epidemic. A local area schedule will probably not differ markedly from the recommended antigen schedule, but it could possibly alter the intervals in the giving of related vaccines or in some other change. The health professionals responsible for immunizing obviously must be familiar with any local adaptation of the administration schedule. Some time intervals for giving the basic vaccines are suggested in the following discussion, but they are not intended to be definitive.

## COMBINING VACCINES

The routine immunizations are usually given as combined antigens. This decreases the number of required injections and improves the efficacy of the vaccine. Combining medications uses the same underlying principle whether it is applied to vaccines or other drugs. Simply stated, the principle is that the combination of medications enhances the effect of each, improving its therapeutic potential and often, therefore, lowering the dosage needed. Pertussis, for example, seems to behave as an adjuvant in its own right and so increases the immune response when combined with diphtheria and tetanus. In another example, with a combination such as MMR (measles, mumps, and rubella), the overall dosage is lower than if each antigen were given individually. Each antigen enhances the immune response of the others.

## THE BASIC OR PRIMARY VACCINES

Discussion of the routine, or basic, immunizations uses as its framework the combinations regularly seen in practice.

*Diphtheria, pertussis, and tetanus* are available individually or combined and as fluids or adsorbed toxoids. There are various trade names or jargon initials used as shorthand descriptions of the combination, depending on the supplier. Diphtheria also comes in varying antigenic strengths, termed **Lf.,** which denotes the amount of toxin equal to one unit of antitoxin. These differing Lf. values give increased flexibility in administering diphtheria vaccine to persons of varying ages and immunization status. For example, the number of Lf. units in the combination vaccine used for primary protection of infants is usually higher than that for adults.

Diphtheria, pertussis, and tetanus antibodies do not cross the placental barrier. This leaves the infant vulnerable to any of these potentially fatal diseases. Pertussis strikes most often in children under age 5 to 6 years, and diphtheria claimed many young lives before the advent of a safe, reliable toxoid vaccine. (The terror and helplessness of parents fighting their children's diphtheria infection in the prevaccine era is vividly captured in the book *Mrs. Mike*, by Nancy and Benedict Freeman.) The spores of tetanus bacteria can live for years in the soil and present an infection hazard. Because of the child's vulnerability, immunization against diphtheria, pertussis, and tetanus is begun in early infancy, usually at 2 to 3 months of age.

The initial series of combined diphtheria, pertussus, and tetanus toxoid is four doses, one month apart. If the vaccinee's history indicates any health concern, such as convulsions, thereby contraindicating the giving of pertussis, the antigens may be used separately. There are many instances where the immunization rationale has to be tailored to the patient: for example, the adult client who will not receive pertussis and who has proof of current tetanus protection, or the family recently emigrated who are not sure just what protection they have. In situations such as these and others, the antigens will often be separated, so a brief note on each is in order.

**Diphtheria** is continued at approximately five-year intervals throughout life following the initial series. If a person requires primary diphtheria immunization and proof of initial series is unavailable, the **Schick test** may be used. This test indicates the level, if any, of existing diphtheria antibodies. Because of the risk of reactions to diphtheria toxoid in adults, the Schick test provides a safe way of determining immune response and testing for hypersensitivity to the inoculating fluid.

The Schick test uses both forearms: the right for the control to test for protein sensitivity, and the left for the test material, which is a dilute diphtheria toxoid. The right, or control, forearm is read 24 hours later, and the left, or test, forearm is read one week later. The Schick test is interpreted as follows:

| Test | Control | Interpretation |
|------|---------|----------------|
| Negative | Negative | Person is immune—no further immunizing needed |
| Negative | Positive | Immune, but sensitive to toxoid |
| Positive | Negative | Not immune and not sensitive—immunize |
| Positive | Positive | Person is a reactor—do not immunize |

If the person is to be immunized, the Lf. and dosage interval will then be decided, taking into account the type of diphtheria toxoid (plain fluid or adsorbed) to be used, the current schedule, and the manufacturer's recommendations.

If no Schick test is used, immunization may be done with a dilute diphtheria toxoid having lower Lf. units to reduce the risk of reactions.

Both methods require boosters at five-year intervals, with the primary series consisting of four doses, each one month apart.

**Pertussis** is mainly a disease of infants and young children, so boosters are usually not given after school entrance at age 5 or 6 years. Even with adequate immunization, it is possible for a youngster to contract pertussis with its typical cough. In these instances, the disease is often less severe and the risk of secondary complications such as convulsions or encephalitis is reduced. The pertussis component of the combined vaccine must be omitted if the child has a history of convulsions. In this case, immunization would be given using combined diphtheria and tetanus vaccines.

**Tetanus vaccine** is continued throughout life; the current recommended booster interval is every 10 years after the initial series. Tetanus toxoid may be given in instances of "dirty" wounds such as abrasions, knife cuts, or machinery injuries, especially if the person is unsure of their immunization history. Administering tetanus toxoid in emergencies and accidents prevents possible tetanus but risks a reaction to the vaccine if boosters are given too often. Tetanus antigen provides excellent immunity, so the disease itself is now rarely seen and public awareness of the risk has diminished. People whose work or hobby, such as carpentry or gardening, exposes them to greater risk must be reminded of their need for protection by teaching them about the disease and stressing the protective rationale. Certain occupations are more at risk for tetanus; these are outlined in Chapter 6.

In summary, the triple combination vaccine of diphtheria, pertussis, and tetanus is begun in early infancy, with a complete primary series usually consisting of four doses. The combination is boosted at age 5 years, before school entrance. From this age on, the pertussis is eliminated and subsequent boosters are with the dual combination of diphtheria and tetanus. The latter two may be given individually if necessary.

The administration of the diphtheria, pertussis, and tetanus combination vaccine is accompanied by teaching parents and adult vaccinees about the vaccine. They should be warned of a possible local reaction at the injection site six to eight hours later. Local reactions are relieved by applying an ice compress to the injection site and giving ASA or Tylenol. Infants and young children may experience a low-grade fever with irritability or sleeplessness the night of the initial injection. Again, ASA or Tylenol in age-appropriate doses will help. Any severe reactions, such as convulsions, must be promptly reported and treated.

A local reaction, even if marked, such as redness and induration at the injection site, does not mean the vaccine should be discontinued, providing there is no systemic or general response. Local and general reactions are discussed in Chapter 4.

Finally, the immunizing must be done only after screening the vaccinee. The **specific contraindication** to the giving of diphtheria, pertussis, and tetanus is a history of convulsions, which may be triggered by the pertussis component. Always keep in mind the general precautions discussed in Chapter 4. Children who are subject to frequent upper respiratory infections need not miss out on needed protection. The common cold is not necessarily a contraindication to immunizing if the child is not acutely ill or running a fever. It may be that waiting until such children are free of colds exposes them to a greater risk of pertussis or diphtheria. Since diphtheria and tetanus protection continues into adulthood, parents should be given permanent records and the significance of the initial series stressed.

**Poliomyelitis** vaccine has two forms, the live (Sabin) or killed (Salk) vaccine. Available in the trivalent or monovalent form, they both have a reported effectiveness of 90%, with protection against the carrier state as well as the disease. The trivalent form is preferred, since it contains three strains of virus. Sabin vaccine is easily administered orally, and immunity is rapidly achieved. The Salk vaccine may be combined with diphtheria, pertussis, and tetanus as a quadruple vaccine. In Canada and some European countries, Salk and Sabin are used interchangeably, with both exhibiting good antigenic properties. In the United States, Sabin vaccine is used, since Salk is no longer available.

The administration schedule is similar to that of diphtheria, pertussis, and tetanus. Polio protection is begun in early infancy (approximately two months of age), and the complete series is three doses of either Salk or Sabin four to six weeks apart, and a fourth dose six to 12 months later. With either vaccine, a booster dose is needed every three to five years to maintain immunity. If Sabin vaccine is used, there must be a minimum four-week interval between the doses of Sabin as well as between the Sabin and any other live vaccine. Sabin is not recommended as a primary series for pregnant women; it is preferable to give Sabin only as a booster following an initial series of Salk injected vaccine.

Both Salk and Sabin vaccines are well tolerated, with few reported reactions. It is safe to tell patients that no reaction is expected; however, this does not preclude checking with the patient on a return visit. Very rarely, about one person in one million given Sabin oral vaccine may show symptoms of a paralytic reaction. The reaction to killed Salk vaccine could be that of allergic sensitivity, but this is also rare.

Salk injectable vaccine is stored and handled in the same way as other biologicals described in Chapter 4. Sabin oral vaccine, however, requires special handling because it is usually shipped frozen and thawed in the refrigerator. Continuous, adequate refrigeration is mandatory; Sabin vaccine deteriorates once it is opened and left at room temperature or exposed to sunlight. This is an instance where the product brochure will spell out the supplier's storage and handling requirements for Sabin. Generally, Sabin must be destroyed if left at room temperature for longer than 12 hours or if there is any vaccine left over after a clinic. Once opened and used, even partially, it must not be returned to the refrigerator.

**Rubella (German measles)** vaccine differs from the triple or quadruple combinations in that the immunization is not given until after the first birthday because the child retains maternal antibodies. Rubella in itself is not a serious disease, but it is tricky to diagnose definitively because of its vague symptoms and fleeting rash. Its greatest threat is to the unborn fetus, especially in the first trimester of pregnancy. The woman may not develop any symptoms of the disease or even realize she has been exposed, but the fetus is vulnerable to the virus if the mother does not have a sufficiently high level of rubella antibodies circulating in her blood. The congenital malformations caused by rubella can be profound, especially in the first trimester, when the sense organs and cardiac tissue are developing. Because of the potential damage inherent in rubella disease, many health agencies are giving priority to rubella programs for both boys and girls aged one to 12 years to increase herd immunity and lower the risk of fetal exposure for pregnant women.

Rubella vaccine is generally well tolerated. Parents or adult vaccinees should be alerted to possible fever or temporary arthralgia in the weeks following inoculation. These reactions are similar to but less severe than those seen in clinical rubella. Of course, the vaccine must not be given to pregnant women. If it is given to postpubertal women, thorough contraceptive counseling must be foremost in the health teaching. Pregnancy must not occur for a full three months after rubella immunization. At present, one injection of the required dose is thought to confer lasting immunity, but ongoing study may show the need for a booster dose.

*Rubella antibodies and the HI test.*   Rubella immunization programs for males of the 12 years and under age group present no particular administration problems. Programs for postpubertal female patients, however, are a different matter because of the pregnancy risk. The question of rubella vaccination for women with "conception potential" is inextricably involved with antibody titer. To protect fetuses effectively from damage, rubella vaccine should be given to the people most at risk of the disease, in other words, the people whose blood, on examination, shows relatively few rubella antibodies. The **low titer,** or level of antibodies in the blood, indicates no immunity and the person is therefore susceptible to the rubella virus. In theory, then, rubella vaccine could be given selectively to those who demonstrated a low titer. In reality, and for practical purposes in community health, the rubella protection program is directed at those under 12 years old and women in the childbearing age group. If the woman is pregnant, her antibody titer will be checked in one of the earliest prenatal visits to a doctor or clinic; even if she is not pregnant, women in this age group should be advised to have their existing rubella antibody titer measured. A single blood sample is checked using the **hemagglutination-inhibition test,** or the **HI test.** The test result is expressed as a ratio in multiples of eight, such as 1:8, 1:64, 1:256, and so on. The accepted ratio indicating immunity is 1:32, with 1:64 preferred. This accepted value is subject to change with local community practice and continuing research into postvaccine HI testing.

What does this ratio mean? A test result of less than 1:32 means the person has probably never had rubella and is therefore susceptible. The ratio of 1:32 is borderline and may also indicate susceptibility. Results greater than 1:32, such as 1:64 or better, indicate previous exposure, and the person is immune. The fetus is also safe if the maternal antibody titer is 1:64 or better and the pregnant woman is exposed to rubella.

*Pregnancy and rubella disease.*　Pregnant women who suspect exposure to possible rubella infection and are unaware of their HI status need prompt care. In this instance, two blood samples are needed, one immediately after contact and the second 14 to 21 days later. (This interval is the incubation period for rubella.) The two samples are tested together at the end of the incubation period and the results compared. If the first sample result is a low ratio (less than 1:32) and the second is high, this indicates recent exposure to rubella with no previous immunity. Since this means the pregnant woman is susceptible to the disease, her fetus also risks viral damage. Depending on the stage of the pregnancy, the possibility of congenital abnormalities exists in such a situation. Further testing, such as amniocentesis, may be advised, with the accompanying moral and ethical dilemma of **therapeutic abortion.** For the couple trying to make a decision, this can be a time of intense personal crisis with perhaps long-lasting ramifications. The ultimate decision regarding the pregnancy must be theirs to make; they will be greatly assisted by a nurse who respects their judgment, offers therapeutic support, and continues contact with the couple in subsequent weeks, regardless of the outcome. Offering continuity of care after the initial crisis is over can be one of the most satisfying aspects of family work in the community.

*Rubeola (red measles)* vaccine, like rubella, is a live vaccine given after the first birthday because of the child's retained maternal antibodies. Some conditions require rubeola immunization before age 1 year: if families live in isolated settlements with infrequent visits by health workers and limited opportunities to immunize, or if the risk of rubeola infection is great and the children are susceptible, as in the case of indigenous Indian families. This early rubeola inoculation must be followed by another dose after the first birthday to ensure a sufficient immune antibody level in the child. Adults do not require rubeola protection because they usually have acquired immunity. As with rubella, an injection after age 1 year is presently felt to confer immunity, but future research may show the need for booster doses.

Rubeola vaccine is usually well tolerated, but parents should be told that children may, occasionally, exhibit a measleslike reaction. This consists of either a rash and/or a temperature. The rash is not as widespread as it is in clinical rubeola, nor is the temperature as high, usually staying below 102°F (39°C).

In addition to the regular screening of the vaccine there are **specific contraindications** for rubeola. The first is sensitivity to eggs, chicken feathers, and the antibiotic neomycin. Since the vaccine is grown in a chick embryo culture medium with neomycin in the base fluid, all these potential allergens are present.

A second specific contraindication involves an interesting relationship between tuberculosis and rubeola. The live measles vaccine causes a temporary depression in tuberculin sensitivity and can result in false-negative readings with the tuberculin skin test. Tuberculin skin testing should be done before rubeola immunization. Children with untreated, active tuberculosis should not be given rubeola vaccine in order to avoid superimposing a side effect of the vaccine on the underlying illness.

Finally, caution is necessary in giving rubeola, with its possible reaction, to children with a history of febrile convulsions. Children known to have had seizures, febrile or otherwise, should be immunized by their family physician.

*Mumps* vaccine is usually given in combination with the two measles vaccines but can be given alone if necessary, with a 30-day interval between the mumps and any other live vaccine.

Experimental and clinical studies are strengthening the argument in favor of simultaneous administration of certain vaccines. It had been suggested in the past that simultaneous administration of live vaccines could cause more serious side effects as well as a diminished antibody response. The recommendation that live virus vaccines be given together or at one-month intervals reflects ongoing investigations into immunity. Mumps live vaccine confers a satisfactory antibody level, although it is not as high as that produced by a natural infection. A single injection is presently thought to be sufficient but, as with other vaccines, immune surveillance continues and may ultimately show the need for a booster. Mumps vaccine is given to children over 15 months of age and susceptible adults.

Contraindications to administration of mumps vaccine are similar to the other live measles vaccines. These include allergy to chicken eggs or feathers, sensitivity to neomycin, and the giving of other live vaccines within one month. Tuberculin testing should also be done before giving mumps vaccine to eliminate a possible false-negative reading due to suppression of tuberculin sensitivity.

Mumps vaccine is usually well tolerated with few reactions. Occasionally, a mild fever may occur and/or parotitis in those previously exposed to natural mumps.

The combined vaccine of rubella, rubeola, and mumps is stored and handled in much the same way as oral polio vaccine. The manufacturer will outline requirements in the product leaflet packed with the vaccine.

## STUDY QUESTIONS

1. The pertussis vaccine is not recommended beyond age
   _____.

2. In the absence of injury, booster doses of tetanus are recommended at intervals of _____ years.

3. After interpreting a Schick test, if you decide to immunize, you are immunizing a person against _____.

4. A vaccine that requires special shipping (i.e., frozen) and handling to prevent deterioration of the product is
   _____.

5. Rubella vaccine is not given until after the first birthday because _____.

6. The major purpose of rubella immunization programs is to
   _____.

7. Pregnancy must not occur for _____ months after rubella immunization.

8. The preferred ratio indicating immunity in an HI test is
   _____.

9. Combined vaccines are presently being used to immunize for _____ and _____.

10. Two contraindications specific to rubeola vaccine are
    _____ and _____.

# BIBLIOGRAPHY

Balfour, H. H., and D. P. Amren. "Rubella, Measles and Mumps Antibodies Following Vaccination of Children." *American Journal of Diseases of Children,* **132**(6), 573–577 (1978).

Bean, J. A., L. F. Burmeister, C. L. Paule, et al. "A Comparison of National Infection and Immunization Estimates for Measles and Rubella." *American Journal of Public Health,* **68**(12), 1214–1216 (1978).

Benenson, A. S., Ed. *Control of Communicable Diseases in Man,* 12th ed. Washington, D.C.: American Public Health Association, 1975.

Brown, M. S. "What You Should Know About Communicable Diseases and Their Immunizations, Part 1, The Three R's." *Nursing 75,* **75**(9), 70–72 (1975).

Brown, M. S. "What You Should Know About Communicable Diseases and Their Immunizations, Part 2, Diphtheria, Pertussis, Tetanus and Polio." *Nursing 75,* **75**(10), 56–60 (1975).

Chow, M. P., B. A. Durrand, M. N. Feldman, et al. *Handbook of Pediatric Primary Care.* New York: Wiley, 1979. Pp. 49–69.

Evans, A. S., Ed. *Viral Infections of Humans. Epidemiology and Control.* New York: Plenum, 1976. Pp. 195–196.

Freeman, B., and N. Freeman. *Mrs. Mike.* New York: Bantam, 1963.

Furesz, J. "Poliomyelitis Outbreaks in the Netherlands and Canada." *Canadian Medical Association Journal,* **120**(8), 905 (1979).

Gangulu, R., and R. H. Waldman. "Effect of Orange Juice on Attenuated Rubella Virus Infections." *Indian Journal of Medical Research,* **66**(3), 359–363 (1977).

Infectious Disease Service. *Immunization and Related Procedures in Infants and Children.* Toronto: The Hospital for Sick Children, 1973.

Kaufman, D. B., W. C. deMendonca, and J. Newton. "Diphtheria-Tetanus Skin Testing." *American Journal of Diseases of Children,* **134**(5), 479–483 (1980).

Kettyls, D. M., M. E. Towell, S. Segal, et al. "Clinical Statement. Rubella (German Measles)." Vancouver, B.C.: Perinatal Program of British Columbia, 1976.

Krugman, S. "Rubella Immunization: Progress, Problems and Potential Solutions." *American Journal of Public Health,* **69**(3), 217–219 (1979).

Marks, M. I., Ed. *Common Bacterial Infections in Infancy and Childhood.* Baltimore: University Park Press, 1979. Pp. 29–31.

Meyer, H. M., H. E. Hopps, P. D. Parkman, et al. "Control of Measles and Rubella Through Use of Attenuated Vaccines." *American Journal of Clinical Pathology,* **70**(1), 128–135 (1978).

Middaugh, J. P. "Side Effects of Diphtheria-Tetanus Toxoid in Adults." *American Journal of Public Health,* **69**(3), 246–249 (1979).

Mortimer, E. A., and P. K. Jones. "An Evaluation of Pertussis Vaccine." *Reviews of Infectious Diseases,* **1**(6), 927–932 (1979).

Nelson, J. D. "The Changing Epidemiology of Pertussis in Young Infants. The Role of Adults as Reservoirs of Infection." *American Journal of Diseases of Children,* **132**(4), 371–373 (1978).

Nichols, E. M. "Atypical Measles Syndrome: A Continuing Problem." *American Journal of Public Health,* **69**(2), 160–162 (1979).

O'Neill, A. E. "The Measles Epidemic in Calgary, 1974–75:The Duration of Protection Conferred by Vaccine." *Canadian Journal of Public Health,* **69**(4), 325–333 (1978).

Shaw, E. B. "Commentary on Immunization." *American Journal of Diseases of Children,* **134**(2), 130–132 (1980).

Vickery, D., and J. Fries. *Take Care of Yourself, A Consumer's Guide to Medical Care.* Reading, Mass.: Addison-Wesley, 1977. Pp. 161–169.

# 6

---

# Immunization
# for Special Needs

When you have successfully completed this chapter, you will be able to:

1. Discuss important management protocols in caring for the health of immigrants and refugees.

2. Describe primary preventative interventions for persons preparing for overseas travel.

3. Counsel persons regarding immunizations recommended due to occupational hazards.

4. Recognize the special immunization needs of two maturational age groups and apply this information in clinical practice.

5. Demonstrate an understanding of the risk of immunizing persons with chronic illness by referring them appropriately.

Community health nurses frequently counsel people who require very different vaccines from those offered in the routine, or basic, immunization programs. Before any inoculations can be given, however, some thorough "detective" work must be done to uncover any previous injections that may be recorded elsewhere, perhaps in another language, or need retrieval from the "memory bank"! It is unsafe to assume that certain antigens have or have not been given; for example, some countries routinely administer typhoid or poliomyelitis vaccines, while other countries do not. Time spent in sleuthing often results in the discovery of documentation of earlier injections; this time spent with the client is also an opportunity for information sharing and teaching.

Although there are many situations that involve the rearrangement or adjustment of antigens for particular needs, this chapter discusses certain groups of people whose requirements are more frequently encountered in practice. These groups are refugees, immigrants, travelers to destinations outside North America, workers at occupational risk for some diseases, senior citizens (aged 65 and over), pregnant women, and people with chronic diseases such as emphysema or diabetes.

## REFUGEES

The term **refugee status** is synonymous with unique health concerns. These families have often suffered extreme deprivation in the weeks and months before a harried departure from home and arrive in their receiving country physically and emotionally exhausted. They have endured, in a short period of time, multiple losses such as occupation, income, country of origin, and ethnic majority, as well as possible separation from, or deaths of, family members. Some of the immediate and urgent priorities of refugee families, such as housing and financial aid, are obviously beyond the scope of this handbook: however, health concerns, such as infectious disease or intestinal parasites, surface quickly and need early attention.

## Reception Clinics

Clinics geared to the unique needs of refugees are specially set up in communities receiving the arriving groups. Refugee reception clinics use a team approach as recognized in public health practice, in delivering health care; such team members include nurses, social workers, physicians, and translators. In contrast to everyday practice, in which there is planning time, the health team's approach and methodology may have to be altered in order to deal effectively with language differences, culture and travel "shock," a large influx of people in a short time period, and a wide range of ailments, some of which will be acute. The reception clinic sorts out the initial priorities such as housing or acute illness, enlists other help for the family as needed, such as diet information from a nutritionist, and, most important, insures ongoing care for the family by instituting a follow-up procedure with the appropriate public health agency in the family's new community.

## Follow-Up Care

The ongoing health needs of refugee families may be similar to, or very different from, other families in their community. The new family from overseas must find dental care and learn about infant feeding and routine immunizations, as do their neighbors. The difference comes in the lack of background knowledge about Canadian and U.S.

health mores and values. Health teaching about immunization will have greater impact if the nurse has acquired basic knowledge about the refugee's country of origin and related health practices. The family itself is the best resource; community health nurses are in an enviable position for learning a great deal about other cultures from sharing and helping the family adjust their health knowledge and habits to North American life. Sharing and learning from each other helps both the refugee family and the nurse. The nurse, when faced with what seems to be reluctance on the family's part regarding a health service such as routine immunization, should recall that the notion of "health for the public" as known in the United States and Canada may be a truly foreign idea for the family. They may be expecting to pay for health services and be unable to do so, so they are hesitant to involve themselves. Refugees do not enjoy the luxury of choosing a country to emigrate to; they have had no opportunity to study our health attitudes, expressions, and practices!

As the newcomers settle in, the children enroll in local schools, increasing the opportunities to work with the families. Immunization with the routine, or basic, antigens (see Chapter 5) is given to the school-aged children after screening. Adults in the family should also be offered the routine antigens of diphtheria (**after** Schick testing; Chapter 5), poliomyelitis, and tetanus.


## SURVEILLANCE

One aspect of follow-up care to refugees that differs from the rest of the community is **surveillance,** or regular supervised monitoring of the family for possible contagious disease. Surveillance is the responsibility of the community health nurse or related health worker from a public health agency following notification from a refugee reception clinic, for example. Surveillance insures that people arriving from countries where infectious diseases are endemic do not develop an infectious disease after arrival and/or transmit that disease to the receiving community. For instance, if cholera was an endemic disease in the family's country of origin and, as refugees, they have not been immunized, the family will be closely watched until the incubation period for cholera is past, about one week. The length of the surveillance period is determined by the incubation period of the questioned disease.

All refugees benefit from a thorough health screening on arrival. They may need particular care for a syndrome peculiar to the area they have come from, but two communicable diseases or conditions are regularly monitored: hepatitis and intestinal parasites. This duo is an endemic fact of life in countries where soil and domestic water supplies are likely to be contaminated with feces and urine. Hepatitis remains difficult to treat; the family members or contacts may be given immune serum globulin, with blood samples taken at intervals to determine the course and contagiousness of the disease. Intestinal parasites are amenable to medication; surveillance involves supervision of the treatment plan and instruction to the family regarding submission of stool samples until no further evidence of infection is found.

Hepatitis and intestinal parasites are not confined solely to refugee families. For this reason, these diseases are discussed fully in Chapters 8 and 10.

Both intestinal parasites and hepatitis require extensive follow-up, and the surveillance period may be uncomfortable for both the nurse and the family if personal judgments interfere. In other words, a nurse educated and practicing in the United States or Canada may associate these diseases with a questionable life-style instead of placing them in the perspective of being common occurrences in tropical and subtropical countries. Also, the family may wonder what all the fuss is about; they have not had to account for themselves in this manner before (i.e., blood and stool samples). Both the refugee family and the health professional need to share their feelings and make the surveillance period a matter-of-fact health procedure—an often fascinating exercise done through an interpreter!

## IMMIGRANTS

Much of the preceding discussion of refugee health concerns applies also to immigrant families except for two significant differences: choice and time. The family in this instance has chosen a new country to call home, has applied for entry, and has had time to fulfil the criteria of the receiving country. Indeed, they may not be admissible until certain socioeconomic and health standards have been met, such as an occupation and disease-free status.

### Reception and Follow-Up Care

Immigrants usually do not need the full services of a reception clinic, since they have met health criteria. They do, however, have many of the same ongoing health concerns as refugee families, such as immunizations, intestinal parasites, and possibly hepatitis or some other illness that, while not excluding them, requires follow-up. Public health agencies are notified in this instance, as they are with refugees.

Like the refugee groups, these families may also be entering from a country where infectious diseases unknown in the United States are endemic; immigrants, however, are expected to provide proof of immunization against diseases present in their original country as well as possible infections in countries through which they will travel en route. Failing proof of immunization status, immigrant families may be immunized on arrival or kept under surveillance until any possible incubation period for a communicable disease is over. The preceding discussion on surveillance also applies to immigrant families.

Once settled, a complete assessment of the family's needs is made, including plans for immunizations for the routine, or basic, antigens. School-aged children are given the vaccines to bring them up to date with their classmates, while the adults are offered poliomyelitis, tetanus, and diphtheria vaccines, the latter given **after** Schick testing (see Chapter 5).

The community health nurse is often one of the first contacts the immigrant family makes in the new country, with potential for much long-range support and teaching for the family. Health workers, in turn, stand to acquire new knowledge about family values and health practices in other different and fascinating cultures.

## OVERSEAS TRAVEL IMMUNIZATIONS

Travel outside North America can present disease risks. Changes in climate, hygiene, food growing and processing,

and questionable water supplies all have disease potential. Some diseases flourish in the tropics, while certain temperate-zone infections may be unknown in warmer climates. Travelers need correct and up-to-date information about the health and hygiene standards in the country of destination.

## Travel Information

One of the most reliable information sources is a public health agency; these offices receive regular bulletins on worldwide disease statistics and overseas immunization requirements. Other information sources are knowledgeable travel agents and airlines, especially if their personnel have actually been to the destination(s) in question. Insight into the practices and environment in the intended country are invaluable for a safe and happy trip.

## Travel Antigens

The guiding principle when counseling travelers is to urge them to leave ample time for administering the needed vaccines. This is based on the rationale that a series of injections spread over several weeks is often required. It confers a higher level of protection if a series can be given at the full recommended intervals instead of squeezing the necessary vaccines into an abbreviated time period. Obviously, the traveler will be much more comfortable and less likely to suffer a reaction. Six months ahead of a projected trip is not too soon, especially if the person has not traveled widely before and is therefore not likely to have current immunization status or if the destination is "off the beaten path."

Countries establish their own **immunization entry requirements;** these are coordinated by the World Health Organization (WHO). These regulations can change, and member countries keep the WHO informed of their requirements. The requirements for entry into a country are dictated by the diseases endemic in that country; for example, Peru and Bolivia require yellow fever immunization, while most European countries do not require any immunizations for entry. There is a difference, too, between immunizations **required** by a country and those that are **recommended.** The former are obligatory, and the traveler may be denied entry without proof of protection; the latter are recommended for travel within the country but are left to the discretion of the tourist and the immunizing nurse. Whether protection is required or recommended depends on the index of infection in the country and the environmental hazards, such as availability of pure food and water. One of the most commonly recommended antigens, for instance, is typhoid vaccine. Although it does not confer a high level of immunity (the traveler must be warned that protection from typhoid is far from 100% with this vaccine), it does afford some margin of safety in countries where typhoid is a possibility. Typhoid vaccine is discussed on p. 101.

## Smallpox Vaccine: Administration and Reaction

Smallpox is no longer a routine or basic immunization because the incidence of disease is virtually nonexistent and vaccination risk outweighs possible disease risk. The worldwide status of smallpox, however, will continue to be monitored for some time and, for this reason, certain countries still recommend or require vaccination. The administration of smallpox vaccine and the expected reaction differ markedly from other antigens and require a more detailed description. Clients receiving an initial smallpox vaccination must have the reaction and the related care clearly explained to them. If a person has had a vaccination within the previous five years, the reaction is barely noticeable.

Smallpox vaccine is a live vaccine made from the closely related cowpox virus. It is introduced into the body by placing a drop of the vaccine on the skin of the deltoid area of the left arm and penetrating through the drop with a sterile needle to make a tiny puncture or scratch. A single "pox" results, with the reaction slowly building from a red bump to a pustule in 10 to 14 days. The pustule gradually dries and a scab forms. This scab finally falls off in about three weeks, leaving a small scar.

This description applies to the **initial** or **primary take,** and this must occur to give immunity. Occasionally individuals, for unique reasons, do not produce a "take" in spite of repeated attempts. Generally, three attempts may be made and, if no primary reaction develops, an appropriate notation should be made on the person's permanent record. If proof of smallpox immunity is required for travel and there is no primary take or the vaccine itself is contraindicated, this person will need an official letter of explanation from a public health agency.

The **significant contraindications** to smallpox are skin conditions such as psoriasis or eczema, and pregnancy. With a reaction consisting of a vaccine-filled pustule, one can visualize the risks of possible infection to broken skin areas if leakage occurs. In fact, all family members must have intact skin to prevent any possible secondary infection from the vaccination. In pregnancy, the virus will cross the placenta, causing possible fetal infection or spontaneous abortion. The other general contraindications apply as well, including the one-month interval between smallpox and another live vaccine.

Booster vaccinations are done every five years and usually do not produce repeated scars. The booster reaction is a small red bump at the site, with no other signs. If the interval has been prolonged, the person should be warned that another primary reaction may occur.

Because the primary reaction of smallpox is pronounced and visible, parents and vaccinees will find a thorough explanation reassuring. The health teaching should include a description of the pustule formation and the length of time involved as well as a reminder to keep the vaccination dry and open to the air to prevent leakage and speed scab formation. This means no swimming or showering while the pustule is present and no occluding bandage.

As the take proceeds, there will be an area of redness around it, and the upper arm will be sore and hot. The vaccinee may feel feverish, have a low-grade temperature, suffer malaise, and complain of a headache at the peak of the reaction, on about the fourteenth day. Young children may lose their appetite for a day or two, and adults may lose a day or two away from work. Both can feel miserable, but cool liquids to drink and age-appropriate doses of ASA or Tylenol will help.

Smallpox vaccination can occasionally produce severe reactions, an inherent risk with this antigen. These marked post vaccination sequelae include encephalitis, generalized eruptions, secondary infection of the vaccination, or accidental autoinoculation. In this last instance, preventive action can be taken to insure that the vaccination site is the upper, outer aspect of the left deltoid area, cosmetic arguments about the scar notwithstanding. This location prevents contact with an adjacent skin surface.

## Related Health Teaching for Travelers: Hepatitis, Malaria, and Intestinal Parasites

Other antigens for overseas travel include cholera, typhus, yellow fever, and plague. Programs for travel immunization are varied and interesting but, because they represent a small and specialized service, they have not been detailed here. Health personnel involved in travel immunization programs will find much information available and will quickly become familiar with the more exotic antigens. There are other nursing responsibilities, however, besides giving vaccines. The top priority in counseling travelers is the aforementioned time allotment: warn potential tourists to seek information early about the country's requirements for entry and suggest they study material about the country and its inhabitants. The pretrip time period is also invaluable in helping the traveler prepare for conditions that are not immunizable, three of which are problematic: **malaria, hepatitis,** and **intestinal parasites.** There are other diseases, of course, that are definite risks in specific countries; these disease risks have to be discussed with individual travelers, but malaria, hepatitis, and intestinal parasites are widespread in many parts of the world; travelers to South America, the Middle East, the Far East, and similar destinations need thorough teaching. Hepatitis and malaria are both significant risks to the traveler who plans to spend a considerable amount of time in an affected country, use indigenous transportation and accommodation, and consume local food and water. Backpacking hostelers, for example, are more at risk than persons on a three-week tour on "the American plan." Health teaching can be tailored to the traveler's needs without being negative and pessimistic, both instead adding to other pretrip plans. Hepatitis etiology and teaching are covered in Chapter 8.

## MALARIA

**Malaria protection,** in the form of control or immunization, continues to elude epidemiologists and others who study this old disease. In some parts of the world malaria has become resistant to traditional drug treatments, and new medications are being used. Since a thorough coverage of malaria requires a text in itself, comments here are confined to the health needs of travelers, with interested readers directed to related material elsewhere.

Malaria protection does exist in the form of drugs taken to prevent or suppress the development in the blood of the host of the causative agent, a parasitic plasmodium. The plasmodium is introduced into the host by the bite of the female *Anopheles* mosquito. The drug does not render the tourist any less tasty to the mosquito but, once bitten, does prevent the reproduction of the plasmodium in the host's bloodstream. Most malaria-suppressant drugs have a synthetic quinine base and, in order to be effective, must be maintained at a sufficiently high blood level. The drug must also be started before entering a malaria-endemic area; again, note the importance of lead time for trip plans. The specific type and amount of medication to be taken is decided by the destination, since the malarial strains differ in their pathogenicity and resistance to medication. Travelers must begin taking their antimalarial drugs seven to 14 days **before** departure, and they must continue to take them for **a full six weeks after** their return. Six weeks is the incubation period for malaria and, as such, needs to be spelled out; travelers back home in Cincinnati or Portland or Toronto can feel a bit foolish taking antimalarial medication, so they must clearly understand this rationale to prevent any late attacks. In addition, pregnancy is not a contraindication for antimalarial drugs. Once in the malaria-endemic country, clients should be further cautioned to cover their arms and legs if outdoors at dusk, which is "prime time" for mosquitoes, use insect repellent profusely, and have mosquito netting tucked in around the bed mattress. Window screens are not sufficient.

## INTESTINAL PARASITES

The third nonimmunizable disease risk for travelers is **intestinal infection** caused by either **giardiasis** and **parasites** or by **worms.** Another intestinal infection, caused by the protozoan amoeba, is a specific risk in certain locations and should be individually counseled. Giardiasis and intestinal parasites are considerably more serious than "turista," the common traveler's diarrhea. **Turista** is simple diarrhea (i.e., loose, frequent stools containing no blood or mucus). It is not an acute illness; the person has no fever and generally feels fine. Turista will gradually abate after three to five days, as the traveler becomes acclimatized. Giardiasis and intestinal parasites, however, both produce symptoms that persist and/or get worse. Nurses counseling travelers should be familiar with the etiology of these two hazards; they are discussed in Chapter 10.

Finally, as well as taking their antimalaria medication, travelers must be instructed to seek treatment for any symptoms that may develop after they are home. These symptoms can include persistent diarrhea, epigastric pain or discomfort, cough, fever, or a general feeling of being run-down. The health care provider must include an assessment of any overseas travel when considering possible causes of ill health.

## Counseling Travelers

Another priority in counseling travelers is a complete and permanent record of their travel antigens, which should be carried with the passport in a safe place, not in their luggage or in a back pocket. The permanent immunization record for travel differs from other records in that it must be stamped by an official health agency (i.e., an agency in a country recognized as a member of the WHO). Travelers should be reminded that this record is needed not only for overseas countries, but also on return to their homes, especially if they have been traveling in a country that has had an outbreak of a particular communicable disease. Clients should be cautioned to keep their permanent record, even if they are doubtful of traveling again; it is proof of immunization and may mean only a booster some time later instead of repeating a series of injections.

Overall, counseling traveling clients for a healthy trip is based on sharing with them some principles of disease transmission. If clients are made aware of how contaminated food and water, as well as insects, can act as vehicles for disease, they can make intelligent decisions with a minimum of worry. Knowing the basic principles will guide them in choosing "covered" foods such as peelable fruits, omitting "naked" foods such as lettuce and other greens grown in questionable soil, and avoiding foods unprotected by screens and/or refrigeration. If the teaching is understood, clients are unlikely to make the common mistake of carefully using distilled water for drinking and then brushing their teeth with tap water!

As a final note, encourage returned travelers to report on their trip to the travel immunization clinic personnel. Such feedback is an excellent check on the subject and quality of the health teaching given before departure.

## OCCUPATIONAL DISEASE RISKS

Certain occupations, by their nature and location, expose workers to the risk of some diseases far more than the general population is exposed to them. Occupations in this category include nurses, police officers, fire fighters, paramedics, ambulance drivers, and related health team members. The disease risks include tuberculosis, tetanus, typhoid, hepatitis B, and possibly diphtheria. Immunization protection is available for diphtheria, tetanus, and typhoid and is usually mandatory for people in these occupations. Diphtheria and tetanus vaccines are covered in detail in Chapter 5, but a note regarding typhoid is in order here, since many readers will have had an obligatory series of injections.

**Typhoid vaccine** may be given alone or in combination with two related subgroups of typhoid, paratyphoid A and

B. This combination, dubbed TAB in immunizing short-hand, can have a third addition of tetanus, or TABT. When given alone or in combination, the initial series is three injections, with a booster every three years. Aside from screening for general contraindications, (Chapter 4), there are no other specific contraindications against the giving of typhoid. Vaccinees often complain of low-grade fever and a feeling of malaise in the evening of the initial injection day, with possible local redness at the injection site. These symptoms are relieved with age-appropriate doses of ASA or Tylenol, and cold compresses on the injection site. Remember to check for reactions with clients returning for subsequent shots in a typhoid series; subsequent injections often do not cause a repeat of the reaction, but they may in some people. Also, since typhoid antigen is one of the most frequent travel immunizations, be sure to check if the prospective traveler's occupation required a previous typhoid series.

At-risk occupations can be protected against **tuberculosis** by bacille Calmette-Guérin (BCG) vaccination. The rationale and criteria for BCG programs differs from the routine antigens and involves tuberculin skin testing before and after BCG vaccination. The vaccination is only one element in the overall picture of tuberculosis; a complete description of tuberculosis disease, health teaching, and BCG vaccination is found in Chapter 15. Understanding the basic process and treatment of tuberculosis will benefit anyone engaged in those occupations at possible risk and assist them in counseling others.

**Hepatitis A** and **B** are related viral diseases. Hepatitis B, formerly called serum hepatitis, is a particular threat to workers in health-related occupations. Both types of hepatitis are discussed in Chapter 8.

# IMMUNIZATION FOR RETIRED CITIZENS

People over age 65 need immunization programs designed for their needs. For example, most people in this age will have an acquired immunity or sensitivity to diphtheria, so this antigen is not recommended, but they do need to keep their poliomyelitis and tetanus protection current. If they are traveling, this is a good opportunity to bring all their immunizations up to date, in conjunction with those required for a trip.

Many retired people enjoy good health, but others are maintained on medication of various types such as digitalis, antihypertensives, and oral diabetic tablets. Screening this age group before immunization must take into account possible medication(s), especially the steroid drugs. It may be many years since the retired vaccinee has had immunization injections, and antigens may also have changed, so health teaching and follow-up regarding reactions is just as vital here as it is with younger clients.

People over age 65 often inquire about injections of **influenza vaccine.** Influenza antigen varies from year to year because it is made to give immunity against the particular strain of influenza virus current in a given autumn and winter. Influenza can be a deadly infection in persons of senior years, especially if they have chronic respiratory or heart disease placing them at greater risk. Many such individuals have an annual "flu shot" to prevent an acute and serious illness.

Influenza vaccine is a live vaccine, made from antigenic material grown in a chick embryo culture. **Specific contraindications,** therefore, are allergy to chicken eggs or feathers, as well as current respiratory infection and corticosteroid therapy. A rare complication following injection of the swine influenza strain vaccine is **Guillain-Barré syndrome,** or infectious polyneuritis, which may affect one person in 100,000. This syndrome can leave the person with permanently damaged motor ability.

In most instances, influenza immunization is done on an individual basis; that is, the person at risk will be assessed and the vaccine will be given by the family doctor, who will be most familiar with the client and any pertinent health history. Occasionally, if the imminent influenza strain is particularly virulent and large-scale infection is a threat, mass public immunization clinics may be indicated. For herd immunity to be effective, these public clinics must be held well in advance of the virus showing up in the community.

## PREGNANCY AND IMMUNIZATION

Pregnancy is a specific contraindication in immunization programs using live vaccines because of the risk of fetal infection or damage from placental crossover. The contraindicated vaccines are smallpox (see this chapter under travel immunization), rubella and rubeola (German and red measles, Chapter 5), and oral poliomyelitis (Sabin). Killed or attenuated vaccines, such as Salk poliomyelitis antigen and diphtheria and tetanus toxoids, do not carry the same risks and may be used for protection. Many of the antigens used for travel immunization are also killed vaccines, such as typhoid and cholera, and so are given to protect the pregnant and traveling client. Overseas travel while pregnant, however, is not always in the woman's best health interests because of other disease risks for which there is little or no protection (see travel antigens in this chapter). A further complication may be the hazard of placental crossover of foreign viruses or bacteria that do not cause severe clinical illness in the woman but can provoke a deleterious response in the fetus; some of the overseas strains of influenza are an example here. Nurses may seem negative counseling pregnant women against overseas travel, but it is sound advice, especially if the intended destination is offbeat or the woman is in the early weeks of her pregnancy. This is also a time when the woman's diet and rest need to be optimal; tiring travel arrangements and strange foods do not help achieve that objective.

## CHRONIC ILLNESS AND IMMUNIZATIONS

Chronic illness in clients of any age necessitates individualizing their immunization protection. Nurses in schools encounter students with chronic illnesses such as cystic fibrosis and diabetes. Elsewhere in the community, antigenic protection may be needed for adults with multiple sclerosis or emphysema. Whatever the situation, such clients are usually not immunized in public health clinics but by their family doctor, who has access to a full health history. The public health clinic may choose to immunize on receipt of an authorizing note from a physician, and the public health agency will authorize by stamp the travel record of anyone immunized by their doctor.

Unless the person with the chronic illness is at special

risk (e.g., an influenza or measles epidemic), they will likely be protected from major communicable diseases by herd immunity.

## STUDY QUESTIONS

1. The length of time a community health worker should observe refugees for contagious diseases endemic to their country of origin depends on the _____ of the disease.

2. Two communicable conditions that must be monitored in families with refugee status are _____ and _____.

3. Immigrants usually require less intensive observation for infectious disease because _____.

4. Contraindications to smallpox vaccination include _____ and _____.

5. The process of scab formation after smallpox vaccine is administered indicates that a _____ has occurred.

6. A one-month interval between smallpox vaccination and other live vaccines is required and is an important reason why community health nurses should encourage _____ _____.

7. Precautions against contracting malaria include travelers taking antimalarial drugs seven to 14 days before departure as well as for a full _____ weeks after their return.

8. Immunization with TAB or TABT can cause reactions including _____, _____, and _____.

9. Unless a large-scale influenza pandemic is imminent, flu vaccine is usually recommended primarily for

   _____.

10. A complication of swine flu immunization is the potential occurrence of _____ syndrome.

## BIBLIOGRAPHY

Abeles, "Tuberculosis in the Foreign Born." *American Review of Respiratory Disease,* **117**(1), 185 (1978).

Ashley, M. J., T. W. Anderson, and W. H. LeRiche. "The Influence of Immigration on Tuberculosis in Ontario." *American Review of Respiratory Disease,* **110**(2), 137–146 (1974).

Barker, W. H., and J. P. Mullooly. "Impact of Epidemic Type A Influenza in a Defined Adult Population." *American Journal of Epidemiology,* **112**(6), 798–813 (1980).

Barrett-Connor, E. "Chemoprophylaxis of Malaria." *Annals of Internal Medicine,* **89**(3), 417–418 (1978).

Barrett-Connor, E. "The Epidemiology of Tuberculosis in Physicians." *Journal of the American Medical Association,* **241**(1), 33–38 (1979).

Benenson, A. S., Ed. *Control of Communicable Diseases in Man,* 12th ed. Washington, D.C.: American Public Health Association, 1975.

Blake, P. A., M. L. Rosenberg, J. B. Costa, et al. "Cholera in Portugal, 1974, I. Modes of Transmission." *American Journal of Epidemiology,* **105**(4), 337–343, (1977).

Breitenbucher, R. B. "Detection and Chemoprophylaxis of Tuberculosis in Southeast Asian Immigrants." *Minnesota Medicine,* **62**(11), 805–806 (1979).

Byrd, R. B., D. E. Fisk, J. N. Glover, et al. "Tuberculosis in Oriental Immigrants—A Study in Military Dependents." *Chest,* **76**(2), 136–139 (1979).

Center for Disease Control. "Health Status of Indochinese Refugees." *The Journal of the National Medical Association,* **72**(1), 59–65 (1980).

Dupont, H. L., G. A. Haynes, L. K. Pickering, et al. "Diarrhea of Travelers to Mexico." *American Journal of Epidemiology,* **105**(1), 37–41 (1977).

Dyer, R., and J. Keystone. "Malaria, a Canadian Problem!" *The Canadian Nurse,* **77**(1), 20–23 (1981).

Enarson, D., M. J. Ashley, and S. Grzybowski. "Tuberculosis in Immigrants to Canada." *American Review of Respiratory Disease,* **119**(1), 11–18 (1974).

Erickson, R. V., and G. N. Hoang. "Health Problems Among Indochinese Refugees." *American Journal of Public Health,* **70**(9), 1003–1006 (1980).

Francis, T. I. "Epidemiology of Viral Hepatitis in the Tropics." *Bulletin of the New York Academy of Medicine,* **51**(4), 501–507 (1975).

Kavet, J. "A Perspective on the Significance of Pandemic Influenza." *American Journal of Public Health,* **67**(11), 1063–1070 (1977).

Keck, J., and P. Swerhun. "Hepatitis B an Occupational Risk." *The Canadian Nurse,* **76**(11), 33–35 (1980).

Monto, A. S., and H. W. Ross. "Swine Influenza Vaccine Program in the Community: Acceptability, Reactions and Responses." *American Journal of Public Health,* **69**(3), 233–237 (1979).

Neumann, H. H. *Foreign Travel and Immunization Guide,* 9th ed. Oradell N. J.: Medical Economics Company, 1980.

Reichman, L. B., and S. Ruggiero. "Tuberculosis Case Finding Among Aliens Who Entered New York City in 1971." *Health Service Reports,* **89**(2), 177–179 (1974).

Rolfe, E. "Many Travel Personnel Lax About Warning Against Risk of Malaria." *Canadian Medical Association Journal,* **119**(9), 497–502 (1978).

Schonberger, L. B., D. J. Bregman, J. Z. Sullivan-Bolyai, et al. "Guillain-Barre Syndrome Following Vaccination in the National Influenza Immunization Program, United States, 1976–1977." *American Journal of Epidemiology,* **110**(2), 105–123 (1979).

Seah, S. K. *Health Guide for Travelers to Warm Climates,* 2nd ed. Ottawa: The Canadian Public Health Association, 1979.

Vogeler, D. M., and J. P. Burke. "Tuberculosis Screening for Hospital Employees. A Five-Year Experience in a Large Community Hospital." *American Review of Respiratory Disease,* **117**(2), 227–232 (1978).

Walzer, P. D., M. S. Wolfe, and M. G. Schultz. "Giardiasis in Travelers." *The Journal of Infectious Diseases,* **124**(2), 235–237 (1971).

Zako, L. R. "Here are Treatment Protocols for Parasite Control in Refugees." *Michigan Medicine,* **79**(20), 359–360 (1980).

# PART III

## COMMUNICABLE DISEASES NOT PRESENTLY IMMUNIZABLE

Part II dealt with the issues facing health workers managing immunization programs in the community, selectively omitting disease etiology because of the primary control represented by antigen immunity. Part III focuses on communicable diseases frequently seen in public health practice for which, at this point, there is no control by immunization. In Part III, basic disease etiology is now needed, since control of infection as well as effective health teaching uses elements of disease characteristics, transmission, and treatment methods. The aim is now secondary prevention.

Part III continues to use the fundamental principles laid out in Part I, and a review of the first chapter would be helpful. The format differs from Parts I and II in that each chapter is organized under the etiological headings of (1) characteristics of infection and clues to diagnosis, (2) responsible organism(s), (3) transmission of the disease, and (4) treatment and control.

**111**

# 7

---

# Chickenpox: The Varicella Zoster Infections

When you have successfully completed this chapter, you will be able to:

1. Recognize the signs and symptoms of infection with the varicella zoster virus in adults and children.
2. Explain how a definitive diagnosis of chickenpox is made.
3. Describe how chickenpox and herpes zoster are transmitted.
4. Instruct families in the care and treatment of children with chickenpox.
5. Institute measures for controlling the spread of herpes zoster or varicella infection.

### *Characteristics of Infection and Clues to Diagnosis*

Chickenpox is one of the mildest of the childhood viral diseases, but it is one of the most contagious. It is seen most often in winter and spring. Chickenpox begins abruptly with a low-grade fever, mild systemic systems such as malaise, and a generalized rash. The rash is first seen as small, discrete, raised red spots. The spots develop into vesicles, which gradually dry up and form a scab. The most prominent diagnostic clue in chickenpox is the presence of all three stages of the skin eruptions at once. For example, on examining a child, the early rash, some vesicles, and some drying crusts will all be seen together and are probably most visible on the torso. The skin rash in chickenpox tends to erupt in crops, which explains the presence of all three stages at any given time.

Chickenpox, in common with other contagious diseases, tends to be cyclical. In other words, the virulence of the virus can alter from year to year, with children being heavily covered with the rash one season and having very few spots the next. Chickenpox is also a worldwide disease, with most people developing an immunity by their teen years. However, adults can be very ill with chickenpox, just as they can be if they contract other diseases usually seen in childhood such as measles or mumps.

Chickenpox is histologically the same virus as **herpes zoster,** or **shingles.** Children can transmit the virus to adults, especially in the grandparent age group, and have it emerge some time later as shingles. The reverse also holds; adults with a zoster infection can transmit the virus to susceptible children, and chickenpox results. Parents and grandparents should be warned to avoid a painful attack of shingles. For instance, grandparents may be exposed if asked to help care for grandchildren ill with the virus or if children are incubating the virus while visiting.

Herpes zoster is a reactivation of the latent phase of the virus. Instead of causing bodywide spot formation, the vesicles now appear in a particular area on the skin, often following a nerve path, and often unilateral. The vesicles are in patches and are smaller and more closely grouped than in chickenpox—hence the name shingles. The most significant diagnostic clues in herpes zoster are recent exposure to the virus and a **signal patch,** or initial outbreak of a group of vesicles. This alerts an examiner to look for subsequent skin outbreaks on following days.

### Responsible Organism

Both chickenpox and herpes zoster are caused by the varicella zoster virus.

### Transmission of the Disease

Chickenpox, or zoster virus, is passed by person-to-person contact and by droplet or airborne secretions. It is also transmitted by contact with clothing or bed linen contaminated with discharge from the vesicles. The scabs, or drying crusts, are not infectious. After exposure, the susceptible child will exhibit the rash seven to 21 days later and will remain contagious until one week after the last crop of vesicles is seen.

As mentioned, the zoster virus can cross generations. The most difficult characteristic of the herpes zoster virus is its ability to remain dormant in the body and flare up as a shingles attack even years later, perhaps related to a period of stress or another illness. A flare-up of this type usually occurs in adults but can affect children.

### Treatment and Control

For those with immunosuppressed conditions, such as children with leukemia or young infants, this virus can cause severe illness. A person of any age in this risk category should not be exposed to the zoster virus. Grandparents should also be protected from a zoster infection by not having them care for their grandchildren with chickenpox at least until the vesicles are dry.

The vesicles and drying crusts can be itchy, and scratching should be avoided to prevent permanent scarring and possible secondary skin infection. Keep the child's fingernails short. Tepid baths with cornstarch or oatmeal added are soothing, as is calamine lotion applied to the spots. Keep children cool; the itching worsens as the skin warms up.

To help control the spread of infection, children should be kept out of school until the vesicles are dry and should be kept away from susceptible contacts. The clothing and bed linen should be washed in hot water and detergent because leakage from the virus-filled vesicles into pajamas and sheets makes these an infection source.

Adults with a herpes zoster infection may suffer considerable pain and discomfort due to the viral infection of the nerve pathways. They often require analgesia for the acute stage.

Repeat attacks of chickenpox are rare because one infection confers long immunity. The possible dormancy of herpes zoster should be remembered, however, when dealing with this virus. In other words, clinical illness may not immediately result from an exposure to the virus. Instead, it may be harbored by the person, usually an adult, for some time before erupting as shingles.

There is an immune serum globulin made from zoster convalescing patients. It is hard to obtain and expensive, but it may be indicated in situations when high-risk individuals have been exposed to the virus.

## STUDY QUESTIONS

1. The incidence of chickenpox is highest in
_____ and _____.

2. The most prominent diagnostic clue in chickenpox is the
_____.

3. The skin rash in chickenpox is probably most visible on
_____.

4. If exposed to a child with chickenpox, a grandparent may
develop _____ or _____.

5. Zoster virus is transmitted by _____,
_____, or _____.

6. After exposure, the susceptible child will exhibit the rash
_____ to _____ days later.

7. One week after the last _____ is seen, a child is
no longer contagious.

8. To help control the spread of infection, children should be
excluded from school until _____.

9. A flare-up of herpes zoster can be a result of
_____.

10. Immune serum globulin may be indicated to prevent a
severe illness in _____.

## BIBLIOGRAPHY

Baringer, J. R. "Latency of Herpes Simplex and Varicella-Zoster
Viruses in the Nervous System." In A. J. Nahmias, W. R.
Dowdle, and R. F. Schinazi, Eds., *The Human Herpesviruses:
An Interdisciplinary Perspective.* New York: Elsevier, 1981. Pp.
202–205.

Benenson, A. S., Ed. *Control of Communicable Diseases in Man,* 12th
ed. Washington, D.C.: American Public Health Association,
1975.

Brown, M. S. "What You Should Know About Communicable Diseases and Their Immunizations, Part 3, Mumps, Chickenpox and Diarrhea." *Nursing 75,* **75**(11), 35–60 (1975).

Brunell, P. A. "Epidemiology of Varicella-Zoster Virus Infections." In A. J. Nahmias, W. R. Dowdle, and R. F. Schinazi, Eds., *The Human Herpesviruses: An Interdisciplinary Perspective.* New York: Elsevier, 1981. Pp. 10–19.

Brunell, P. A., L. H. Miller, and F. Lovejoy. "Zoster in Children." *American Journal of Diseases of Children,* **115**(4), 432–437 (1968).

Frey, H. M., S. P. Steinberg, and A. A. Gershon. "Diagnosis of Varicella-Zoster Virus Infections." In A. J. Nahmias, W. R. Dowdle, and R. F. Schinazi, Eds., *The Human Herpesviruses: An Interdisciplinary Perspective.* New York: Elsevier, 1981. Pp. 351–362.

Parrish, J. A. *Dermatology and Skin Care.* New York: McGraw-Hill, 1975. Pp. 67, 219–220.

Shore, S. L., and P. M. Feorino. "Immunology of Primary Herpes Virus Infections in Humans." In A. J. Nahmias, W. R. Dowdle, and R. F. Schinazi, Eds., *The Human Herpesviruses: An Interdisciplinary Perspective.* New York: Elsevier, 1981. Pp. 267–288.

Takahashi, M., Y. Asano, H. Kamiya, et al. "Active Immunization for Varicella-Zoster Virus." In A. J. Nahmias, W. R. Dowdle, and R. F. Schinazi, Eds., *The Human Herpesviruses: An Interdisciplinary Perspective.* New York: Elsevier, 1981. Pp. 414–431.

Zaia, J. A. "Clinical Spectrum of Varicella-Zoster Virus Infection." In A. J. Nahmias, W. R. Dowdle, and R. F. Schinazi, Eds., *The Human Herpesviruses: An Interdisciplinary Perspective.* New York: Elsevier, 1981. Pp. 10–19.

# 8

---

# Hepatitis

When you have successfully completed this chapter, you will be able to:

1. Recognize the clinical signs and symptoms of hepatitis A and B.
2. Explain how the responsible organisms in hepatitis A and B are transmitted.
3. Understand the laboratory diagnostic tests for hepatitis A and B.
4. Describe the treatment and control measures for hepatitis A and B.
5. Identify populations or groups at special risk for contracting hepatitis A and B.

Hepatitis is an acute communicable disease affecting the liver; it is endemic in many parts of the world, including the United States and Canada. Community health workers are involved in the teaching and follow-up care with patients and their families and must also be aware of their own occupational risk (related disease risks in health and other occupations are discussed in Chapter 6).

Hepatitis is classified as **A** or **B,** depending on the causative viral agent. There is also, it seems, a third type of hepatitis that does not fit neatly into either the A or B category. This third type is simply called **non-A, non-B** hepatitis and, although it seems to be a posttransfusion type of hepatitis, it is different than hepatitis B, formerly called serum hepatitis. Much study is directed into learning more about all three types of hepatitis, since they all carry the attendant risk of liver damage. Hepatitis A and B will be discussed in turn.

## HEPATITIS A

### Characteristics of Infection and Clues
### to Diagnosis

**Hepatitis A** is the modern name for the older term **infectious hepatitis.** Hepatitis A, in the acute disease, will cause symptoms of nausea, fever, malaise, and abdominal pain to appear suddenly with no clear prodromal period (the time between exposure to the virus and the disease developing). Often, the person feels vaguely unwell and run-down for several days before more acute symptoms develop, or the vague symptoms persist for some days or weeks and then disappear. This latter situation is typical of a subclinical case of hepatitis A; the person may not seek health care and so is unaware of the infection. Depending on the "dose," or exposure to the virus, and the age and health of the person, hepatitis A can vary from such a subclinical picture to a serious illness.

In acute hepatitis A, the symptoms are followed in three to 10 days by jaundice. The patient will notice dark-colored urine and perhaps pale or clay-colored stools. They may also complain of abdominal pain or tenderness, caused by an enlarged liver, and an almost total lack of appetite. In fact, the sight or smell of food may cause a patient to experience increased nausea.

Acute hepatitis A will run its course in about four to six weeks, depending on the severity. In common with other viral diseases, such as infectious mononucleosis (Chapter 9), people recovering from hepatitis A may feel depressed and complain that it is taking them a long time to get their energy back. They should be encouraged not to push themselves into activities that overtire them and to pay particular attention to a high-quality diet. A protracted convalescence of more than a few weeks needs further investigation to rule out any other illness.

**Diagnosis** of hepatitis A is made by clinical examination, with special attention paid to any history of overseas travel within the previous three months. Hepatitis A is widespread in tropical countries, and the U.S. or Canadian traveler is particularly susceptible; the local population develops an immunity to the virus.

Definitive diagnosis must rule out any other cause of the acute abdominal symptoms and the jaundice, such as a malignancy, or a gallbladder obstructed with gallstones. Laboratory diagnosis includes taking blood samples for serological testing of the **serum transaminase levels.** These enzymes, serum glutamic-oxaloacetic transaminase (SGOT) and serum glutamic-pyruvic transaminase (SGPT), will be markedly elevated from an SGOT normal of 10 to 40 U/cc, and an SGPT normal of 6 to 36 U/cc. A specific blood serotype test is not yet available for hepatitis A, and this is a current area of research.

### Responsible Organism

Hepatitis A is caused by a virus. It has only recently (1973) been clearly identified by electron microscopy. The hepatitis A virus is small and shaped like a cube. Most cubed viruses are similar in size, but this one is not and varies considerably in size. (Viral characteristics are discussed further in Chapter 13, under the topic of herpes infections.) The virus resists killing by heat and acids, but it is susceptible to formalin and chlorine, the latter at the same dilution (one part per million) as that required for domestic water supplies.

### Transmission of the Disease

Hepatitis A is spread by the **fecal-oral route.** The virus is excreted in the feces and, if allowed to contaminate food and water, sets up a chain of infection. Urine and blood, including menstrual blood, also frequently contain the virus.

Laboratory study will show the virus in stool samples, providing the samples are taken before the appearance of jaundice. Once the jaundice is apparent, the numbers of viruses present in the stools drop to an undetectable level. As in other infectious diseases, the prodromal period of hepatitis is the most contagious.

Travelers are at risk for two reasons. First, if the destination is one where hepatitis A is widespread, it is difficult to avoid exposure. Second, many countries have inadequate hygiene measures for safe disposal of sewage; the result is fecal contamination of food and water.

Once exposed, symptoms may take up to three months to appear; the average incubation period is about one month. Repeat bouts of hepatitis are not common, indicating that an immunity develops to the virus. How long this immunity lasts is not precisely known.

### Treatment and Control

Control of hepatitis A is by sanitary disposal of sewage and thorough hand washing, especially after toiletting. Patients with active hepatitis A must take care not to expose others by any possible contamination of household articles by feces, urine, or blood. Isolation technique is not required if personal hygiene and sewage are adequate.

For travelers to endemic countries and for close household contacts, there is **immune serum globulin (ISG)** available that will prevent or ameliorate the disease. For long-term exposure to possible hepatitis, as in prolonged travel or occupational risk, the ISG may be repeated two to three times a year. ISG is a passive protection conferred by the presence of antibodies "pooled" in the product that provide a temporary immune cover for an exposed, and therefore susceptible, person. Because the duration of the immune cover is transitory, the ISG needs frequent boosters (two to three times a year) if exposure is prolonged.

## HEPATITIS B

### Characteristics of Infection and Clues to Diagnosis

**Hepatitis B** is the now commonly accepted name for serum hepatitis. It has increased in incidence due to the drug subculture and the increased use of blood and related products. Hepatitis B has a slower onset than hepatitis A; the symptoms (anorexia, fatigue, abdominal pain, nausea, possible vomiting) are the same but do not appear as suddenly. People with hepatitis B may be afebrile and can be suffering from a subclinical infection. In a fully developed infection, however, patients may complain of joint pains, and jaundice does develop some days later, as in hepatitis A. Another similarity is that the prodromal phase is the most contagious. In both instances of hepatitis, patients may not realize that they have been exposed or that they are, in turn, now exposing others to a hepatitis infection. The severity of hepatitis B infection is, like A, related to the dose of viral exposure and the health and age of the host person, but with added risk represented by specific occupational hazards. The latter are discussed under transmission of this disease.

Hepatitis B infection can linger for many weeks and become a chronic infection. Since there are other long-term illnesses of the liver causing related symptoms of impaired hepatic function, long-term hepatitis B needs to be differentiated from these in order to help the patient and control the spread of hepatitis infection.

**Diagnosis** of hepatitis B is clearer than that of hepatitis A because there is a definitive blood test available. The test involves laboratory examination for both a specific hepatitis B surface antigen, called **HBsAg,** and a serum antibody, called **HBsAb.** A positive HBsAG indicates current exposure and infection with hepatitis B; a positive HBsAb indicates earlier exposure. In other words, HBsAg measures the immediate body response to an invading organism by ascertaining the production of a specific antigen; HBsAb will measure the existence of antibodies present as a result of previous exposure to the infection. These serological tests give a quick and accurate diagnosis. Speed is often essential in hepatitis B to pinpoint an infection source and limit exposure of susceptible people.

Liver function testing (SGOT and SGPT) will also be done as part of the diagnostic rationale. Normal values for the tests are given in the discussion of hepatitis A.

### Responsible Organism

Hepatitis B is caused by a virus. The causative virus particle consists of the inner antigen core (the HBcAg) and the outer antigen present on the surface of the virus (the HBsAg). This virus particle, or "package," is typical for hepatitis B and is called the **Dane particle.**

### Transmission of the Disease

Hepatitis B is spread by exposure to infected blood and related blood products such as plasma, packed cells, and serum. The virus is also carried in saliva, semen, and urine. Hepatitis B is further transmitted by exposure to any mechanical devices used in administering blood and blood products such as needles and intravenous equipment and to renal dialysis machinery. Such transmission routes obviously place nurses, laboratory workers, police officers, ambulance drivers, and paramedics at a greatly increased risk of exposure to, and infection by, hepatitis B. Protection for these occupations is discussed under treatment and control.

Because hepatitis B is also transmitted through semen and saliva, there is risk of infection from these sources. For this reason, an increased incidence is seen in groups of people with multiple sex partners. There may also be transmission between spouses if one is carrying the HBsAg. Dentists are at risk if their patient is HBsAg positive.

Tracing the transmission of this disease is made more difficult by the presence of hepatitis antigen (HBsAg) in the blood of many otherwise well people. This is one of the many questions surrounding hepatitis B that is under investigation. One answer may be that the circulating HBsAg is a response to previous subclinical infection with hepatitis B. It is not clear why some people succumb to the infection and others do not when exposure was apparently the same. Obviously, however, the circulating HBsAg offers protection against repeated exposure and infection.

### Treatment and Control

Acute hepatitis B infection will run its course in four to six weeks. During this time, the treatment is usually conservative and supportive, such as bed rest and a high-quality diet. Because hepatitis is a viral infection, antibiotics are of little use and are usually not indicated, and there are no other specific drug treatments. The person recovering from a hepatitis B infection will be serologically monitored to determine the course of the disease, and the necessary teaching to prevent transmission of further infection will be provided. Liver function tests (SGOT and SGPT) will be repeated, and the person may return to work as these approach normal values.

**Patient health teaching** is a large element in the control of hepatitis B. Patients with active disease should not be in contact with possible transmission agents such as blood and its products, laboratory equipment, renal dialysis units, immunization procedures, or the like. Patients will need support and encouragement through the course of the infection and explanation of the laboratory studies. If the person remains HBsAg positive, they will need to assume responsibility for their sexual contacts, especially if the patient has multiple partners. Such a situation requires informed consent on the part of the partner; that is, they need to know that the other person has a possibly transmissable disease and make their decision based on that knowledge.

Convalescing patients must also be encouraged to carry through with the laboratory work and follow-up visits to their doctor to insure a return to health. Hepatitis B can become chronic; in addition, there seems to be an increased risk of developing a liver malignancy. Patients must be informed of their health status and blood test results during the active and convalescent stages of hepatitis.

Because the serological tests in hepatitis B are so specific, they can be used to screen contacts of patients and others who may have been exposed to possible infection. If a person reports a suspected exposure, their blood may be quickly checked for HBsAg and HBsAb. On a repeat check one to two weeks later, an upswing in HBsAg value will indicate recent exposure to the virus.

Controlling the spread of hepatitis B with ISG is not effective as it is with hepatitis A. There is an experimental **hyper-immune globulin** (high in anti-HB antibodies) available, but its use is not recommended because it is felt it may increase the number of carriers in the population.

A new development promises control of hepatitis B. A vaccine has been formulated and its widespread use is imminent. Immunization protection against the virus will then be possible, greatly reducing the hazard of infection for at-risk occupations as well as for the public. Soon public health workers will have another powerful tool in their fight against disease.

## STUDY QUESTIONS

1. Hepatitis A is spread by the _____ route.
2. _____ are particularly susceptible to hepatitis A infections.
3. The incubation period for hepatitis A is _____ to _____ months.
4. Acute hepatitis A will run its course in about _____ to _____ weeks.
5. ISG provides _____ protection for a person exposed to hepatitis A.
6. Hepatitis B is now the commonly accepted name for _____.
7. The initial symptoms of hepatitis B include _____, _____, _____, _____, and _____.
8. Nonparenteral spread of hepatitis B can occur through exposure to _____.
9. Hepatitis B is most contagious before the onset of _____.
10. Infection with hepatitis B can be diagnosed by a blood test for _____.

## BIBLIOGRAPHY

Alcoff, J. "Testing for Viral Hepatitis." *The Journal of Family Practice,* **11**(7), 1029–1035 (1980).

Bauer, D. "Preventing the Spread of Hepatitis B in Dialysis Units." *The American Journal of Nursing,* **80**(2), 260–261 (1980).

Benenson, A. S., Ed. *Control of Communicable Diseases in Man,* 12th ed. Washington, D.C.: American Public Health Association, 1975.

Berkow, R., Ed. *The Merck Manual,* 13th ed. Rahway, N. J.: Merck Sharp and Dohme Research Laboratories, 1977.

Corey, L., and K. K. Holmes. "Sexual Transmission of Hepatitis A in Homosexual Men. Incidence and Mechanism." *The New England Journal of Medicine,* **302**(8), 435–438 (1980).

Crovari, P., and S. De Flora. "Epidemiological Distribution and Significance of Anti-HBs." *Developments in Biological Standardization,* **30,** 302–328 (1975).

Denes, A. E., J. L. Smith, S. H. Hindman, et al. "Foodborne Hepatitis A Infection: A Report of Two Urban Restaurant-Associated Outbreaks." *American Journal of Epidemiology,* **105**(2), 156–162 (1977).

Dienstag, J. L. "Toward the Control of Hepatitis B." *The New England Journal of Medicine,* **303**(15), 874–876 (1980).

Froesner, G. G., U. Sugg, and W. Schneider. "Half Life of Transfused Anti-HBs." *Developments in Biological Standardization,* **30,** 316–319 (1975).

Gardner, P. S., and C. R. Howard, Eds. *Diagnostic Methods in Viral Hepatitis.* New York: Alan R. Liss, 1978.

Gerety, R. J., E. Tabor, R. H. Purcell, et al. "Summary of an International Workshop on Hepatitis B Vaccines." *Journal of Infectious Diseases,* **140**(4), 642–648 (1979).

Gridon, A. J., and R. V. Rosvoll. "Reporting Transfusion-Associated Hepatitis." *Transfusion,* **20**(1), 108–109 (1980).

Hindman, S. H., T. E. Maynard, D. W. Bradley, et al. "Simultaneous Infection With Type A and B Hepatitis Viruses," *American Journal of Epidemiology,* **105**(2), 135–139 (1977).

Hoofnagle, J. H. "Prevention of Type B Hepatitis." *Gastroentology,* **76**(6), 183–185 (1979).

Hoofnagle, J. H., R. J. Gerety, and L. F. Barker. "Hepatitis B Core Antigen and Antibody." *Developments in Biological Standardization,* **30,** 175–185 (1975).

Hooper, R. R., C. W. Juels, J. A. Routenberg, et al. "An Outbreak of Type A Viral Hepatitis at the Naval Training Center, San Diego: Epidemiologic Evaluation." *American Journal of Epidemiology,* **105**(2), 148–156 (1977).

Kelkar, S. S., and R. K. Mahajan. "Hepatitis B Antigen-Carriers. A Two and a Half Year Follow-Up." *Indian Journal of Medical Research,* **66**(3), 353–358 (1977).

Levy, B. S., J. Mature, and J. W. Washburn. "Intensive Hepatitis Surveillance in Minnesota: Methods and Results." *American Journal of Epidemiology,* **105**(2), 127–134 (1977).

Norris, C. "Hepatitis: How to Avoid Infection." *Dental Management,* **17**(3), 36–42 (1977).

Polakoff, S., and W. d'A. Maycock. "Anti-HbAg Immunoglobin After Inoculation Injuries." *Developments in Biological Standardization,* **30,** 329–334 (1975).

Segal, H. E. "Hepatitis B Antigen and Antibody in the U. S. Army. Prevalence in Health Care Personnel." *American Journal of Public Health,* **66**(7), 667–671 (1976).

Szmuness, W., M. I. Much, A. M. Prince, et al. "On the Role of Sexual Behavior in the Spread of Hepatitis B Infection." *Annals of Internal Medicine,* **83**(4), 489–495 (1975).

Szmuness, W., C. E. Stevens, E. J. Harley, et al. "Hepatitis B Vaccine: Demonstration of Efficacy in a Controlled Clinical Trial in a High-Risk Population in the United States." *The New England Journal of Medicine,* **303**(15), 833–841 (1980).

Zuckerman, A. J. "Towards the Conquest of Hepatitis B." *Nature,* **287**(5782), 483–484 (1980).

# 9

---

# Infectious
# Mononucleosis

When you have successfully completed this chapter,
you will be able to:

1. Recognize the signs and symptoms of infectious
   mononucleosis.
2. Explain how definitive diagnosis of infectious mononucleosis is made.
3. Describe the transmission of the Epstein-Barr virus.
4. Instruct individuals and families as to the treatment and control of infectious mononucleosis.
5. Counsel patients during the convalescent period
   to avoid serious sequelae and recurrence of the
   disease.

*Characteristics of Infection and Clues
to Diagnosis*

Infectious mononucleosis, commonly referred to as infectious mono, or just mono, is an acute viral disease with a

wide range of clinical expression. Depending on the virulence of the virus and the susceptibility of the exposed person, it may produce an acute, bedridden illness or simply a period of feeling weak and tired. There are many gradations between those extremes and, although infectious mono is seldom fatal, it can be protracted and debilitating, making the person susceptible to other infections, such as pneumonia.

The most frequent signs and symptoms are fever, lymphadenopathy, sore throat, fatigue, and malaise. There may be a generalized skin rash, and about half the people affected develop enlarged spleens. About 10% of patients also have enlarged livers, while some have both spleen and liver affected.

Definitive **diagnosis** requires laboratory examination of the patient's blood. With infectious mono, the virus causes a change in the number and quality of the **mononuclear lymphocytes,** or white blood cells. There is also a specific antibody produced in response to the virus. On examination of the blood, there will be an abnormal number of white blood cells, and many will be seen in an immature stage of development. The antibody produced that is diagnostic for infectious mono is the **Paul-Bunnell-Davidsohn** antibody (**PBD**), and a positive PBD test is considered confirmation of the disease.

### Responsible Organism

Infectious mono is caused by the **Epstein-Barr (EB)** virus. This virus is related to the herpes simplex virus, which causes cold sores, but it is serologically distinct.

The EB virus is also implicated in **Burkitt's lymphoma,** a malignancy seen in parts of Africa and China. There is no evidence to suggest, however, that having a severe case of infectious mono increases the risk of developing cancer.

### Transmission of the Disease

Infectious mono is transmitted by person-to-person contact, usually by kissing. Since it is most often seen in older children and young adults, it has been nicknamed the "kissing disease" or the "student's disease." The virus can be carried in the nose and throat for weeks after an infection and may be further transmitted by airborne droplet secretion. There is also the possibility of infection through blood transfusion from undiagnosed cases or someone in the carrier state.

### Treatment and Control

Infectious mono is a self-limiting disease and will run its course in two to five weeks if uncomplicated. Treatment is usually symptomatic, with acetylsalicylic acid (ASA) used for fever and malaise and extra rest recommended. Antibiotic therapy is indicated only if the person has a secondary or related infection such as a streptococcal sore throat.

Infectious mono may take as long as six weeks to manifest itself but, after exposure, the average incubation period is about two weeks. Isolation of the ill person is not indicated.

While convalescing, patients with liver or spleen enlargement should use caution as they resume activity. They must avoid strenuous athletics and heavy lifting.

Feeling depressed is one of the more subtle complaints voiced by people recovering from infectious mono. They often feel it is taking far too long to feel well again, and they have trouble getting their energy level and morale back. Such complaints must be carefully investigated, especially because these patients are often young adults with hectic schedules and perhaps questionable health practices, such as inadequate nutrition.

## STUDY QUESTIONS

1. The extent of ill health experienced by a patient with infectious mono depends on _____ and _____.

2. About 10% of patients with mono exhibit _____, and half of the people affected develop _____.

3. More frequent signs and symptoms are _____, _____, _____, _____, and _____.

4. A positive _____ test is diagnostic for infectious mono.

5. Infectious mono is caused by the _____ virus.

6. This virus causes a change in the number and quality of _____ blood cells.

7. This virus can be carried in the _____ and _____ and can be transmitted for _____ (time) after an infection.

8. The age groups in which infectious mono is most often seen is _____ and _____.

9. The average incubation period of infectious mono is _____.

10. Isolation of the patient _____ required in cases of infectious mono.

# BIBLIOGRAPHY

Benenson, A. S., Ed. *Control of Communicable Diseases in Man,* 12th ed. Washington, D.C.: American Public Health Association, 1975.

Chang, R. S. *Infectious Mononucleosis.* Boston: G. K. Hall, 1980.

Chang, R. S., L. Rosen, and A. Kapikian. "Epstein-Barr Virus Infections in a Nursery." *American Journal of Epidemiology,* **113**(1), 22–29 (1981).

Connelly, R. R., and B. W. Christine. "A Cohort Study of Cancer Following Infectious Mononucleosis." *Cancer Research,* **34**(5), 1172–1178 (1974).

Epstein, M. A., J. R. North, and A. J. Morgan. "Approaches to the Prevention of Epstein-Barr Virus Infection." In A. J. Nahmias, W. R. Dowdle, and R. F. Schinazi, Eds., *The Human Herpesviruses: An Interdisciplinary Perspective.* New York: Elsevier, 1981. Pp. 432–440.

Evans, A. S. "Epidemiology of Epstein-Barr Virus Infection and Disease." In A. J. Nahmias, W. R. Dowdle, and R. F. Schinazi, Eds., *The Human Herpesviruses: An Interdisciplinary Perspective.* New York: Elsevier, 1981. Pp. 172–183.

Henle, W., and G. Henle. "Clinical Spectrum of Epstein-Barr Virus Infection." In A. J. Nahmias, W. R. Dowdle, and R. F. Schinazi, Eds., *The Human Herpesviruses: An Interdisciplinary Perspective.* New York: Elsevier, 1981. Pp. 31–34.

Merigan, T. C. "Immunosuppression and Herpes Viruses." In A. J. Nahmias, W. R. Dowdle, and R. F. Schinazi, Eds., *The Human Herpesviruses: An Interdisciplinary Perspective.* New York: Elsevier, 1981. Pp. 309–316.

Miller, G. "Oncogeneisis by Epstein-Barr Virus." In A. J. Nahmias, W. R. Dowdle, and R. F. Schinazi, Eds., *The Human Herpesviruses: An Interdisciplinary Perspective.* New York: Elsevier, 1981. Pp. 228–236.

Pearson, G. R. "Epstein-Barr Virus: One or a Family of Viruses." *Cancer Research,* **34**(5), 1237–1240 (1974).

Pearson, G. R., and L. Aurelian. "Immunology of Herpes Virus-Associated Cancers." In A. J. Nahmias, W. R. Dowdle, and R. F. Schinazi, Eds., *The Human Herpesviruses: An Interdisciplinary Perspective.* New York: Elsevier, 1981. Pp. 297–308.

Shore, S. L., and P. M. Feorino. "Immunology of Primary Herpes Virus Infections in Humans." In A. J. Nahmias, W. R. Dowdle, and R. F. Schinazi, Eds., *The Human Herpesviruses: An Interdisciplinary Perspective.* New York: Elsevier, 1981. Pp. 267–288.

# 10

---

# Parasitic Conditions and Infections

When you have successfully completed this chapter, you will be able to:

1. Recognize the characteristic signs and symptoms of three communicable skin infestations.
2. Explain how the responsible organisms are transmitted.
3. Apply treatment and control measures for the eradication of outbreaks of lice, ringworm, and scabies.
4. Identify intestinal parasitic infections seen in U.S. and Canadian communities.
5. Institute preventative measures for treatment and control of parasites.

The term parasite is defined as a plant or animal living in or on another organism, usually to its detriment. This aptly describes the infections discussed here, since each represents an in or on situation producing various degrees of harm to the human host. The topics are pediculosis (nits and lice), ringworm, scabies, and intestinal parasites (pinworms, roundworms, and giardiasis). There are two related conditions also included for ease of reference: toxoplasmosis, and *Toxocara canis* and *T. cati.*

# PEDICULOSIS

### *Characteristics of Infection and Clues to Diagnosis and Responsible Organism*

The term **pediculosis** means infestation of clothing or the hairy parts of the body by the human louse. Lice will, therefore, infect the hair of the head, axillae, or pubis. The body louse will be found in the inner seams of clothing, especially if the garments are bulky, heavily layered, dirty, or infrequently changed.

On examination, a health worker may see both lice and nits, the latter being the eggs deposited on the hair shaft or in the clothing seams. Lice are small (2–5 mm, or ⅛ in.), pale brown insects that move rapidly when disturbed. The nits, however, cling tenaciously to the hair or garment and cannot be shaken loose or easily dislodged. They resemble flakes of dandruff, but it is this firm attachment that alerts the examiner. When inspecting the hair, it is common to find only the nits, and these are frequently seen behind the ears and along the base of the hairline. Because the lice bite the scalp, the person often complains of an unusually itchy head.

Pediculosis knows no social or economic boundaries. Although it may be a greater health problem in areas of overcrowding and poor sanitation, it is found in all communities and, in fact, is enjoying ill-found popularity in some!

### Transmission of the Disease

Because of their mobility, lice will migrate from one infested head to another or from one person to another if contact is close and toilet articles such as combs and brushes are shared or headwear is exchanged.

### Treatment and Control

The nits hatch in about one week and are capable of reproducing in approximately two weeks. The person is therefore contagious until all the lice and nits are destroyed. Anyone is susceptible, and repeated infestations can occur if control measures are not thoroughly implemented. Lice and nits in the scalp hair are treated by dusting malathion powder (lindane) into the hair, taking care to cover all areas, or by shampooing with a product called Kwell (in Canada, Kwellada) until no further signs of infestation are seen.

There is a risk of further irritation of the scalp with these insecticides if the skin is already excoriated by bites or scratching. Even if the scalp is intact, these agents may cause irritation in certain skin types. They should be used with care and probably not repeated more often than twice a week. There is also concern about the absorption of these products through the skin, but, at this time, they are the most readily available and inexpensive treatments. If discontinuing use of either of these insecticides is indicated, the remaining nits may be removed using a special fine-toothed, or nit, comb.

**Controlling outbreaks** of pediculosis in group settings such as schools or camps involves excluding and treating infected people and consistently checking their contacts. Inspection of schoolchildren or other groups should be done on a regular basis to prevent any possible epidemic. Lice are infamous nomads! Children should be taught not to share head coverings and hair articles.

Parents may react angrily if their child is excluded from school with pediculosis that did not originate with them. They may be unaware that this condition is now widespread and interpret it as a derogatory comment on their care. It helps to explain that pediculosis is a community problem and that no one is immune. It also helps if parents are kept up to date with other related school health issues such as dental care or immunization programs; many schools include such information in regular bulletins taken home by students. In this manner, a less acceptable issue such as pediculosis may be put into better perspective.

The **pubic,** or **crab, louse** closely resembles the head louse in appearance and habit. Besides infesting the pubic hair, these nits may be seen on the eyelashes or the hair of the axilla. Transmission of pubic lice and nits is usually by intimate contact. Treatment is by dusting affected areas with malathion powder (lindane).

The **body louse** is one of the classic health problems of overcrowded and unhygienic conditions. Its characteristics are similar to hair and pubic lice, but now the insecticide should be dusted over the entire body. The clothes and bed linen should be boiled in soapy water, dry-cleaned, or burned.

Of these three lice, the head louse is the most common.

# RINGWORM

### Characteristics of Infection and Clues to Diagnosis

**Ringworm** of the body takes its name from the typical ring-shaped skin lesion caused by the infection spreading outward and leaving a center area of apparently normal skin. The outside perimeter of the lesion may be reddened and flaky, while the overall appearance may be dry and scaly or moist with small vesicles. In the early stages, before the expanding ring is clearly visible, the patch of affected skin may be confused with eczema, psoriasis (see Chapter 13), the signal patch of herpes zoster (see Chapter 7), or neurodermatitis. A careful history noting possible sources of infection helps eliminate these; once the typical ring is seen, there is little doubt.

**Athlete's foot,** caused by the same group of fungi, is a frequent complaint. Instead of the ring formation, the fungus produces an often intense burning and itching of the skin on the feet. The skin may be deeply cracked or fissured, or scaly in appearance, particularly between the toes. All of this is made worse by athletic activity (hence the name), which makes the feet hot and damp with perspiration. Some of these infections are deep seated and difficult to eradicate.

### Responsible Organism

Ringworm is caused by one or more of a group of fungi called the dermatophytes.

### Transmission of the Disease

Ringworm can be transmitted by direct contact with an infected person or by indirect contact through contamination of hair articles, shower stalls, towels, headrests on seats, and the like.

### Treatment and Control

The typical lesion will appear within two weeks after contact and is treated by topical application of a fungicidal ointment. In severe cases, it may be necessary to use a systemic oral medication called griseofulvin. Control extends to thorough cleaning of pools, showers, and gymnasium apparatus with a fungicidal agent at regular intervals. People with active lesions should, of course, be excluded from showers and gyms, but this is difficult in practice. As a preventive control measure, and also because of the widespread occurrence of athlete's foot, public pools install shallow troughs, filled with a fungicidal solution, arranged so that swimmers are expected to walk through them going to and from the pool and showers. If more people were aware of this or had ever suffered from athlete's foot, there would be fewer people stepping over the troughs!

For the treatment of athlete's foot, topical fungicidals, either cream or powder, are used with griseofulvin taken orally in stubborn instances. Encourage the person to wear pure cotton socks (since synthetic materials do not absorb perspiration), change them frequently, and boil them between wearings. Shoes, particularly running shoes, should be dried completely before wearing and dusted with fungicidal powder. The feet should also be washed and dried carefully and exposed to the air by wearing sandals if possible.

There are two other locations subject to fungus infections: the **scalp** and the **nails. Scalp ringworm** may be missed at the outset until the lesion is large enough to be seen in the hair. It causes the hair to become dry and brittle and fall out, sometimes resulting in permanent baldness. The fungus in this instance can be present in domestic pets and cattle; the stray kitten or puppy brought home is the traditional clue. Scalp ringworm is quickly diagnosed by an ultraviolet light called the **Woods light,** which causes the lesions to fluoresce. Since scalp ringworm can be widespread among children in particular, some communities routinely screen schoolchildren using the Woods light.

**Ringworm of the fingernails** or **toenails** is a stubborn infection. Fortunately, it is virtually noncontagious even with intimate contact, but it is a discouragingly chronic affliction. The nails become dry, fragile, and corrugated in appearance and surrounding skin can also be affected. This fungal infection is a truly unappealing condition and if the fingernails are affected, the sufferer is forever explaining to onlookers.

The fungus infections of the feet, scalp, and nails share the same characteristics and treatment as body ringworm with the exceptions as noted. In all instances of fungal conditions except that of the nails, teaching should alert people to the routes of transmission to prevent possible contamination and spread.

## SCABIES

### Characteristics of Infection and Clues to Diagnosis

The common name for **scabies** is the itch, and it certainly does! Classically, scabies infection is described as making reddened lines, or tracks, on the skin, but this is not always seen. Often the skin will have a more generalized rashlike appearance, with patches of itchy and broken skin. The itching can be intense, and the condition is made worse by scratching. Scabies can be confused with other skin conditions such as eczema or psoriasis (see Chapter 13), but a careful history noting the progression of the lesions as well as the typical itching will rule out other skin problems. In many instances, scabies infections do not fit the textbook locations of the flexor surfaces of the arms or between the fingers, instead they may be seen on the upper chest, around the waist, or the back and buttocks.

### Responsible Organisms

Scabies is caused by the female itch mite, *Sarcoptes scabiei,* which burrows under the skin and lays eggs. This burrowing causes the tracking or lines and the itching. The mite can be diagnosed microscopically, but clinical signs usually suffice.

### Transmission of the Disease

Scabies is passed by direct contact with an infected person or by indirect contact such as infected clothing or bed linen. Families or groups can infect each other for weeks and months, creating a stubborn and discouraging infection. Anyone can contract scabies with sufficient exposure, but the incidence is higher with overcrowding, transiency, sexual promiscuity, and poor hygiene.

### Treatment and Control

After exposure, the appearance of the itching skin lesions varies. It may take several weeks before the individual is aware of a skin problem. Once infected, the person is contagious until the treatment is completed. The treatment program begins with a hot bath and thorough scrubbing of the skin. After this the whole body, with the exception of the face and head, is swabbed with either a 5% solution of benzyl benzoate or a 1% solution of Kwell (or Kwellada). The solution should air dry on the skin. Bed linen and pajamas should be changed. The next day, the person has a cleansing bath and another change of nightwear and bedding. The infected clothing and sheets should be boiled, or washed in hot water and detergent. Nonwashable garments should be dry-cleaned. Some families or individuals may require close nursing supervision to ensure conscientious follow-through of this program and halt further spread of the infection.

Patients should be alerted to the fact that itching may still persist even if the treatment was correctly carried out. This is primarily due to related sensitization of the skin; it should gradually disappear over the next few days. Scabies of long duration can become entrenched in the skin and may require a second identical course of treatment if marked skin improvement and healing is not seen within a week or two.

Since it is almost impossible not to scratch the eruptions, there is a risk of secondary skin infection. Fingernails should be kept short and clean, and the broken areas should be closely watched, especially with children. Patients should be instructed to seek further dermatological advice if healing does not progress following correct treatment.

Scabies control requires exclusion from school or other groups. All family members or those similarly exposed should be checked for possible infection and concurrent treatment initiated if necessary.

## INTESTINAL PARASITES

**Helminths,** or **intestinal worms,** are more common in U.S. and Canadian community practice than we might like to believe. **Enterobius,** or **pinworms,** are the most frequently encountered, but **ascaris** or **roundworms** are present in our population and are more dangerous than the pinworm. The third intestinal parasite is **giardia,** which, although not a helminthic but a protozoan infection, is included because it is an intestinal infection with a significant index of infection in our communities.

### Enterobiasis (Pinworms)

#### *Characteristics of Infection and Clues to Diagnosis*

As the name implies, these intestinal worms are roughly the length and diameter of a straight pin. They resemble short pieces of white thread when seen in the stool. Because of the migratory habit of the female pinworm, there is anal irritation and itching. In severe infestations in girls, this irritation and inflammation may affect the vulval area. The age groups with the highest incidence are young school-age and preschool children.

Many people still believe that children have pinworms when they grind their teeth at night, are overly active, or scratch the inside of their nose. These are fallacies; the best clue is the anal scratching.

Pinworms are quickly and definitively diagnosed. Instruct the parent to apply a piece of transparent adhesive tape to the child's anus first thing in the morning before bathing or going to the toilet. The eggs laid by the female worm at the anal opening will be present on the skin and cling to the sticky tape. They can then be seen microscopically.

### Responsible Organism

The enterobic helminth is the cause of pinworms. It is found only in humans. The worms mature in the small intestine, and the female worm migrates through the anus to lay her eggs on the surrounding skin. The life cycle of the worm is three to six weeks. The eggs live only a few hours after leaving the intestine, but the person remains a source of infection until all the mature female worms are destroyed.

### Transmission of the Disease

Pinworms are transmitted by the anal-to-hand-to-mouth route. In other words, the child scratches the anal area and picks up eggs on the hands or under the fingernails. The eggs are then ingested orally as a result of the frequent hand-to-mouth contact in this age group, and they hatch in the intestine. Young children frequently reinfect themselves and others in this manner. Adults caring for children are also susceptible. If pinworms are diagnosed, the whole family should be treated in order to break the cycle of infection.

Pinworms may be indirectly transmitted by the use of shared clothing and bed linen.

### Treatment and Control

Pinworms are destroyed by the use of an oral antihelminthic agent. These are sold under various trade names and often may be purchased by parents from a reputable pharmacy. Parents and children should be warned that some of these products cause a marked change in the color of the stools. As mentioned, the whole family should be treated simultaneously. In the case of a class of affected children, the teacher should also take the medication.

The infection is **controlled** by thorough hand washing, especially after defecation. This is one reason, along with diminishing hand-to-mouth contact, that incidence decreases with age. Children should be taught that a proper hand washing includes soap, hot water, and a scrub. Frequent changes of underwear and bed linen and the use of hot water in laundering will also help prevent and control pinworm infection.

## Ascariasis (Roundworms)

### Characteristics of Infection and Clues to Diagnosis

The **ascaris,** or **roundworm,** also lives in the small intestine. We generally associate this helminth with the tropics, but it is often seen in the southern United States and frequently in immigrant and refugee populations. This parasite can be present in large numbers in the intestinal tract and excreted in the stool. It is about the length and diameter of a garden earthworm, so is clearly visible. The infection initially causes no clear symptoms, but the sufferer gradually feels less well and complains of gastrointestinal pain as the worm burden increases. Malnutrition and anemia often accompany heavy infestation; the worms may be coughed up as well as fecally excreted. **Diagnosis** is quickly made in either instance.

### Responsible Organism

The human roundworm, or ascaris, is the responsible parasite.

### Transmission of the Disease

The ascaris is not passed directly from person to person but by vehicles such as raw fruits and vegetables previously contaminated by soil containing the eggs (i.e., the soil is first infested by feces containing the eggs). The eggs use the intermediate environment of the soil to reach a developmental stage that makes them capable of living in humans. Once the eggs are ingested, they hatch out in the intestine to become larvae; in the larval stage, they use the blood and lymph systems to migrate through the intestinal wall to vital organs such as the lungs or liver. This infection of vital organs is the particular danger with roundworm infections. Once established, the ascaris continues to reproduce and proliferate in organs and intestine.

Young children and the elderly are especially prone to developing acute symptoms related to respiratory or hepatic involvement, but anyone with a heavy ascarid infection is also at risk.

### Treatment and Control

Ascariasis is treated with an antihelminthic preparation containing piperazine. As with enterobiasis (pinworms), the person is treated until all mature female worms are destroyed (i.e., the stool samples are normal). The worm reaches a mature reproductive age about six to eight weeks after the eggs are ingested and will live for 12 to 18 months.

**Control** of roundworm infection obviously means preventing contamination of soil by feces containing the eggs. This means adequate sewage treatment and disposal, or privies built in such a way that they cannot overflow or fill with water and infect the surrounding areas. Correct hand washing is another control measure, and children should be taught not to eat food that has dropped on the floor or the ground. Persons arriving at North American destinations from ascaris endemic areas should be screened for the parasite by submitting stool samples. Roundworm infection is not usually a factor in refusing immigrant status for health reasons, but community health nurses must be aware of the treatment and control aspects because those families may be under health surveillance until they are rid of the parasite. Such surveillance may be confusing and upsetting for families already trying to adjust to new customs and a strange language, especially if ascarid infection was common in their country of origin. They may have difficulty understanding our concern, and their family beliefs and practices should be respected as much as is healthfully possible. (Refer to Chapter 6 for further discussion of refugee and immigrant health concerns.

# Giardiasis

### Characteristics of Infection and Clues to Diagnosis

**Giardiasis** causes gastrointestinal symptoms such as diarrhea, abdominal bloating, and foul-smelling stools. It is chiefly a risk to travelers, especially those touring Russia, but is also endemic in the United States. It is not sporadic or self-limiting, as is the common traveler's diarrhea, or turista, but it is prolonged if not treated and can result in dehydration, weight loss, and debilitation. It can be confused with ulcerative colitis, so a thorough health history and careful differentiation is needed.

### Responsible Organism

The cause of giardiasis is a flagellated protozoan, the *Giardia lamblia*. The protozoan confines itself to the intestine but can cause inflammation and possible damage to the intestinal mucosa in severe cases.

### Transmission of the Disease

Giardiasis is transmitted by the fecal-oral route or by water contaminated by infected feces. There is a significant problem with a carrier state in giardiasis, and these individuals may be a transmission source.

*Treatment and Control*

Giardiasis is treated with metronidazole (Flagyl), an anti-protozoan agent. Even with treatment, patients should be warned that the infection can recur. Travelers need information about avoiding foods and water where fecal contamination is possible; this extends to avoiding the use of tap water for hand washing or toothbrushing. **Control** also extends to screening immigrants if they are entering from an area of high incidence, such as Russia.

Finally, two related parasitic conditions, each needing a brief comment, are toxoplasmosis and *Toxocara canis* and *T. cati.*

## Toxoplasmosis

**Toxoplasmosis** is caused by a protozoan parasite, *Toxoplasma gondii,* which is becoming better known and understood. Cats excrete the cysts of the protozoa in their feces; the family cat poses a risk to the pregnant woman who cleans out the cat's litter tray. Even though the adult woman may not be clinically ill with the parasite, the infection crosses the placenta and damages the fetus. This fetal harm takes a variety of forms, including congenital malformations and possible intrauterine death. The litter tray chore should be delegated to a nonpregnant family member, preferably male. There is some controversy about the family cat even sharing the house with a pregnant woman. The best health teaching would discourage contact between the two.

## Toxocara canis and Toxocara cati

**T. canis** and **T. cati** are larval stages of a nematode carried by domestic dogs and cats. The eggs of the nematode are passed in the animal's stools and infect the soil. Children contract the infection by playing in sandboxes used by cats or by eating contaminated dirt. (Strange as it seems, some children do go through a dirt-eating stage in their development!) Home sandboxes should be covered when not in use, and cat and dog feces should be removed from lawns and play areas. Kittens and puppies should be wormed before being sent to new homes. Children must be reminded that puppies and dogs should not lick their faces and that they must wash their hands thoroughly after outside play in the dirt or after handling dogs and cats.

## STUDY QUESTIONS

1. A method of preventing a possible epidemic of pediculosis or head lice is to _____.

2. Eradication of head lice includes the use of shampoos or powders containing _____.

3. The antibiotic used in oral treatment of ringworm infections of the skin, including athlete's foot, is

_____.

4. Transmission of ringworm can be through direct contact with an infected person or indirectly by _____.

5. Scabies is caused by the impregnated female itch mite _____, which is transmitted from one person to another by _____.

6. The best indication that a patient has scabies is _____ skin lesions commonly misdiagnosed as psoriasis.

7. Pinworm infection is controlled by thorough hand washing, especially after _____.

8. Ascaris is not passed directly from person to person but by _____, such as unwashed fruit and vegetables.

9. Health teaching regarding giardiasis transmission for travelers includes ⎯⎯⎯⎯⎯⎯⎯.

10. A systemic protozoan disease transmitted by cats that can cause fetal malformations or death is ⎯⎯⎯⎯⎯⎯⎯.

# BIBLIOGRAPHY

Belle, E. A., T. J. D'Souza, J. Y. Zarzour, et al. "Hospital Epidemic of Scabies: Diagnosis and Control." *Canadian Journal of Public Health,* **70**(2), 133–135 (1979).

Benenson, A. S., Ed. *Control of Communicable Diseases in Man,* 12th ed. Washington, D.C.: The American Public Health Association, 1975.

Brown, H. W. *Basic Clinical Parasitology,* 4th ed. New York: Appleton-Century-Crofts, 1975.

Craun, G. F. "Waterborne Giardiasis in the United States: A Review." *American Journal of Public Health,* **69**(8), 817–819 (1979).

Eaglstein, W. H., and D. M. Parlser. *Office Techniques for Diagnosing Skin Disease.* Chicago: Year Book Medical Publishers, 1978.

Eveland, L. K., M. Kenney, and V. Yermakov. "The Value of Routine Screening for Intestinal Parasites." *American Journal of Public Health,* **65**(12), 1326–1327 (1975).

Gemrich, E. G., J. G. Brady, B. L. Lee, and P. H. Darham. "Outbreak of Head Lice in Michigan Misdiagnosed." *American Journal of Public Health,* **64**(8), 805 (1974).

Hand, J. "Lice: How to Break the News Gently." *RN,* **42**(11), 27–29 (1979).

Kanaaneh, H. A., S. A. Rabi, and S. M. Badarneh. "The Eradication of a Large Scabies Outbreak Using Community-Wide Health Education." *American Journal of Public Health,* **66**(6), 564–567 (1976).

Kolff, C. A., and R. Sánchez. *Handbook for Infectious Disease Management.* Menlo Park, Calif.: Addison-Wesley, 1979. Pp. 203–206, 214.

Kuntz, R. E. "Parasites of Children in the United States." *Pediatric Nursing,* **5**(6), 12–17 (1979).

Malarkey, L. M. "Ridding School Children of Parasites—A Community Approach." *Maternal Child Nursing,* **4**(6), 363–366 (1979).

Medical News. "Intestinal Parasites Ranging Far Afield in United States." *The Journal of the American Medical Association,* **239**(26), 2756 (1978).

Melton, L. J., S. A. Brazin, and S. R. Damm. "Scabies in the United States Navy." *American Journal of Public Health,* **68**(8), 776–778 (1978).

Oberle, K., and A. Wildgrube. "Intestinal Helminths." *The Canadian Nurse,* **77**(2), 14–17 (1981).

Orkin, M., H. I. Maibach, L. C. Parish, et al., Eds. *Scabies and Pediculosis.* Philadelphia: Lippincott, 1977.

Parrish, J. A. *Dermatology and Skin Care.* New York: McGraw-Hill, 1975. Ch. 8.

Smith, D. E., and J. Walsh. "Treatment of Pubic Lice Infestation." *Cutis,* **26**(6), 618–619 (1980).

Thacker, S. B., S. Simpson, T. J. Gordon, et al. "Parasitic Disease Control in a Residential Facility for the Mentally Retarded." *American Journal of Public Health,* **69**(12), 1279–1281 (1979).

Wachtel, D. "Consultation—Preventing Scabies Outbreaks." *Nursing 79,* **9**(6), 68–70 (1979).

Watson, T. G., R. S. Freeman, and M. Staszak. "Parasites in Native People of the Sioux Lookout Zone, Northwestern Ontario." *Canadian Journal of Public Health,* **70**(3), 179–182 (1979).

Welch, N. M. "Recent Insights Into the Childhood 'Social Diseases'—Gonorrhea, Scabies, Pediculosis, Pinworms." *Clinical Pediatrics* (Philadelphia), **17**(4), 318–322 (1978).

Wright, R. A., H. C. Spencer, R. E. Brodsky, and T. M. Vernon. "Giardiasis in Colorado: An Epidemiologic Study." *American Journal of Epidemiology,* **105**(4), 330–336 (1977).

# 11

## Salmonella

When you have successfully completed this chapter, you will be able to:

1. Recognize the signs and symptoms of bacterial food poisoning.
2. Explain how food and beverages become contaminated with salmonella.
3. Apply epidemiological measures in uncovering the source of infection in outbreaks of salmonella food poisoning.
4. Describe the treatment of salmonellosis.
5. Instruct individuals and groups in methods for preventing outbreaks of salmonellosis.

Bacterial food poisoning can ruin a pleasant evening out, a family picnic, or a joyful celebration. Many instances of food poisoning go unreported and uninvestigated, perhaps due to a lack of knowledge or a reluctance to discredit someone's hospitality. How frequently the saying is heard: "Oh, I ate something that didn't agree with me!" Perhaps it also did not agree with others who ate the same food, especially if they were very young, elderly, or already partially incapacitated by a chronic illness.

Food can be contaminated by any one of a number of bacteria, such as salmonellae, staphylococci, the clostridii botulinum and welchii, and others. Salmonella is the most frequent cause of food poisoning and is a reportable illness; for these reasons, it will be the focus of this chapter. Many of the principles and criteria involved in the epidemiology of food poisoning are similar; understanding salmonella infections will give a working baseline for the others as well. In addition, many excellent references are available on the other related types of bacterial food poisoning.

### Characteristics of Infection and Clues to Diagnosis

The W.'s and the T.'s, two couples who were good friends, had planned their evening out together for some time. They were going to a German-style *Oktoberfest* to enjoy each other's company, the food, and the oompah music. They had a wonderful time; everyone said that they had especially enjoyed the European-style sausages with sauerkraut. The next day, four very uncomfortable people compared notes; their symptoms varied in intensity, but all were ill with severe abdominal pains and diarrhea. Mr. W. and Mrs. T. have also had episodes of vomiting early in the morning. They agreed that, since they had all been at the same function and eaten the same food, it was a likely case of food poisoning and not any other infection, such as influenza. The couples also agreed to report their illness and their suspicions to the local public health office; they later learned that the sausage meat had been contaminated with salmonella, which thrived in the temperature of the steam tray. The serving arrangements kept the sausages warm, not hot; the temperature was insufficient to kill the bacteria and, in fact, fostered its proliferation.

Some of the foods most frequently implicated in this type of bacterial food poisoning are raw and insufficiently cooked meat, poultry, unpasteurized milk and milk products, and eggs, especially in cracked shells. The W.'s and the T.'s could have become ill from eating the cream-filled pastries, too!

Once ingested, the bacterial contaminant will cause signs and symptoms to develop in 12 to 36 hours; for example, an evening meal will cause illness early the next morning. The diarrhea, vomiting, abdominal cramping, and low-grade fever gradually subside as the day goes on. Depending on the "dose" of bacteria eaten and the age and health of the host person, the reaction can vary from fairly mild, to acute distress with possible hospitalization, to a fatal illness. The sometimes severe abdominal pain must be distinguished from a surgical emergency such as appendicitis or an intestinal obstruction.

**Diagnosis** of salmonellosis, or salmonella food poisoning, is made by noting clinical symptoms and their onset, in conjunction with a food recall for the previous 24 hours. Laboratory culture of stool samples will yield typical growth of the organism and is a definitive diagnostic aid.

### Responsible Organism

The salmonella are a large group of rod-shaped, or bacillus, bacteria. They are not spore forming but are equipped with flagella, which make them motile. There are subgroups in the large salmonella family, and immune response is type-specific. In other words, a person can have antibodies present against one strain, or serotype of salmonella, but fall ill from another.

The hundreds of differing strains of salmonella are dealt with in practice by naming them after the location of the outbreak. Depending on where groups of people were infected, there are salmonella strains, or serotypes, bearing names such as *S. Miami, S. Newport,* and *S. London.* Two salmonella serotypes are particularly infamous because they cause typhoid and paratyphoid fever: *S. typhi* and *S. paratyphi.* These two serotypes keep their names regardless of location.

The salmonella group are called **gram-negative** by bacteriologists. This means that the organism does not retain the Gram's stain and becomes virtually invisible when the microscope slide is washed with alcohol. In order for it to be seen and studied, a counterstain must be applied; this second stain is retained by the bacilli, making them visible under the microscope.

Salmonella bacilli produce an **endotoxin,** or substance within the cell, that is released when the organisms die. This means that a sufficient number of the bacilli must be ingested and die in order for the endotoxin level in the intestine to be high enough to produce symptoms. This makes the onset of illness later than for toxic food poisoning such as staphylococcus, which produces an **exotoxin**, a substance outside the cell. Exotoxins are then immediately available after ingestion of the contaminated food and cause symptoms two to four hours after eating. The onset of symptoms, therefore, is important when assessing the client.

Salmonella is a widespread bacterium, present in the intestines of most farm animals, poultry, and domestic pets.

Salmonella can also linger for periods in the human intestines, producing a temporary carrier state, even if the person has not had an attack of this food poisoning. Since it continues to be excreted from the animal or person, there can be a fecal-to-hand or water-to-mouth route of cyclical recontamination.

The salmonella family will resist cold temperatures, even to freezing and below. They remain quiescent in any contaminated food until that food is thawed or warmed. As the temperature increases, so does the reproduction of the bacteria; body temperature is close to the ideal climate for salmonella. In order to kill the bacteria, the temperature must be "high enough, fast enough, and held for a long enough" time period, as, for example, in the pasteurization process, or in bringing meat to a proper temperature quickly to cook it, followed by prompt refrigeration if not served immediately. Keeping food warm instead of piping hot encourages the growth of salmonella, particularly if the holding period is prolonged.

### Transmission of the Disease

Food can be inoculated with salmonella in a variety of ways, beginning at the slaughterhouse. Since most animals harbor the bacillus in their intestine, the carcass can be infected by slaughter practices. Rigid guidelines and inspection of such practices is set out under food preparation bylaws, but, because of its widespread and invasive nature, salmonella is a tricky organism to supervise effectively.

The butcher and the purchaser are the next links in the chain; the purchaser unknowingly brings salmonella into the home on the surface of the raw meat. Other items in the grocery bag may also carry salmonella, not just on the surface, but within the product, such as meat pies, sausages, the body cavity of poultry, and the eggs picked up as a bargain because of their cracked shells.

Salmonella-free food can be contaminated by flies that have been in contact with feces containing the bacillus. Domestic pets may carry the organism on their paws or in their fur. Baby turtles, bought as children's pets, are another salmonella source. People may be unaware that they harbor the organism in their own intestine and inoculate the food by preparing it with unwashed hands. Thorough hand washing, preferably with a nailbrush, and most definitely after going to the bathroom, is urged for all food handlers, whether in the home or in a public restaurant.

### Treatment and Control

Salmonellosis varies in its severity, depending on the "inoculated dose" of the bacillus. For this reason, treatment of the type of food poisoning is tailored to the outbreak. Usually, supportive care (bed rest, clear fluids) is the main treatment. If the attack is severe, hospital care may be needed, with intravenous therapy for rehydration. Antibiotics are usually not indicated, except for very short periods, since they run the risk of developing a resistant strain. What may be a home care case of food poisoning for a young and healthy person could be a hospital visit for someone who is elderly, very young, or already ill. In turn, members with salmonellosis can infect others in the family, so they should not knowingly expose them to a disease risk.

**Controlling** salmonella means intercepting the path of transmission by methods such as adequate hand washing and preventing fly and animal contamination of food in the home. Cooking temperatures must be brought to high heat quickly (not hours of barely simmering) and the food must either be served very hot, to kill the bacteria along with the endotoxin, or promptly refrigerated. Leaving warm foods standing on counters to cool is an unhealthy practice.

Foods that may contain salmonella within (instead of on the surface) such as meat pies, rolled roasts, and poultry, must be cooked until the internal temperature is high enough to kill any bacteria. A meat thermometer inserted into the middle of such foods is an excellent idea. Stuffing, or poultry dressing, should not be left inside the bird after the initial hot meal; remove it from the body cavity and refrigerate it separately. Because poultry is frequently the cause of salmonellosis, the body cavity should not be filled ahead of time; this practice creates an environment ripe for proliferation of the bacillus.

Home-canned meat is another example of possible salmonella contamination within the food. Preserving meat in the home runs the risk of contamination by other organisms more deadly than salmonella; *Clostridium botulinum* is one. It is to be discouraged, but if families feel there is no alternative, they need thorough instruction from an allied member of the health team, such as a nutritionist or food inspector. With any home canning of meat or vegetables, a pressure cooker must be used, not the open kettle method.

**Note:** *C. botulinum* spores have been found as a contaminant in unpasteurized honey. Infants given pacifiers dipped in unpasteurized honey run the risk of this serious to fatal infection.

A further salmonella control measure is to ensure that people who have had the infection are removed from food preparation or serving. It is not known exactly how long a person remains an infection threat by harboring salmonella in the intestines, but the period can be weeks or months.

People who have suffered food poisoning may be asked to submit stool samples to ensure that they are free of the organism.

Common sense and good hygiene practices will protect foods and consumers from most bacterial contamination. This is certainly true for salmonella, which poses no threat with adequate preparation and storage facilities for food. Nurses can raise family awareness of possible dangers by teaching about salmonella and food contamination in general.

## STUDY QUESTIONS

1. The _____ bacterium is the most frequent cause of food poisoning.

2. The incubation period of this bacterial food contaminant is _____.

3. The symptoms associated with this type of food poisoning are _____, _____, _____, _____, and _____.

4. The natural origin of this bacteria is the intestines of _____ and _____.

5. Salmonella gains access to foods through _____, _____, and _____.

6. Foods causing this type of food poisoning have either been _____ or _____.

7. People can be severely ill with salmonella poisoning, especially _____, _____, or _____ people.

8. The use of a _____ ensures that the center of the food is cooked thoroughly.

9. *C. botulinum* spores are found as a contaminant in
_____.

10. Food poisoning outbreaks are usually recognized by the
_____.

## BIBLIOGRAPHY

Benenson, A. S., Ed. *Control of Communicable Diseases in Man,* 12th ed. Washington, D.C.: American Public Health Association, 1975.

Center for Disease Control. "Salmonellosis in the United States, 1968–1974." *The Journal of Infectious Diseases,* **133**(4), 483–486 (1976).

France, G. L., D. J. Marmer, and R. W. Steele. "Breast-feeding and Salmonella Infection." *American Journal of Diseases of Children,* **134**(2), 147–152 (1980).

Horwitz, M., R. A. Pollard, M. H. Merson, et al. "A Large Outbreak of Foodborne Salmonellosis on the Navajo Nation Indian Reservation, Epidemiology and Transmission." *American Journal of Public Health,* **67**(11), 1071–1076 (1977).

Jawetz, E., J. L. Melnick, and E. A. Adelberg. *Review of Medical Microbiology,* 12th ed. Los Altos, Calif.: Lange, 1976. Pp. 208–211.

Kazemi, K., G. Gumpert, and M. I. Marks. "Clinical Spectrum and Carrier State of Nontyphoidal Salmonella Infections in Infants and Children." *Canadian Medical Association Journal,* **110**(11), 1253–1257 (1974).

Kolff, C., and R. Sanchez. *Handbook for Infectious Disease Management.* Menlo Park, Calif.: Addison-Wesley, 1979. Pp. 120–121.

Levy, B. S., and W. McIntire. "The Economic Impact of a Food-borne Salmonellosis Outbreak." *The Journal of the American Medical Association,* **230**(9), 1281–1282 (1974).

MacCready, R. A., J. P. Reardon, and I. Saphra. "Salmonellosis in Massachusetts." *The New England Journal of Medicine,* **256**(24), 1121–1128 (1957).

Marks, M. I., Ed. *Common Bacterial Infections in Infancy and Childhood.* Baltimore: University Park Press, 1979. Pp. 105–106.

Roueche, B. *Annals of Epidemiology.* Boston: Little, Brown, 1967.

Saphra, I., and J. W. Winter. "Clinical Manifestations of Salmonellosis in Man. An Evaluation of 7779 Human Infections Identified at the New York Salmonella Center." *The New England Journal of Medicine,* **256**(24), 1128–1134 (1957).

Taylor, J. *Bacterial Food Poisoning.* London:The Royal Society of Health, 1969.

Trickett, J. *The Prevention of Food Poisoning.* Cheltenham, England: Stanley Thornes, 1978.

Zaki, M. H., G. S. Miller, M. C. McLaughlin, et al. "A Progressive Approach to the Problem of Foodborne Infections." *American Journal of Public Health,* **67**(1), 44–49 (1977).

# 12

---

# Sexually Transmitted Diseases

When you have successfully completed this chapter, you will be able to:

1. Identify the signs and symptoms of sexually transmitted disease (STD) infections.
2. Know the organisms responsible and the diagnostic methods for the STDs commonly found in clinical practice.
3. Know the incubation periods for the STDs discussed in this chapter.
4. Describe the treatment and control measures for the sexually transmitted diseases.
5. Prevent the spread of STDs by means of client counseling and health education.

The intimate areas of human relationships are an integral part of community nursing. Therapeutic interactions with families acknowledge that sexual expression and functioning are, in turn, an intrinsic component of overall health functioning; thorough and empathetic assessment and planning with clients at all stages in the life cycle include sexual functioning as part of the total health assessment. Clients suffer a disservice and health workers a credibility "demotion" when sexuality is sidestepped with the excuse of embarrassment to one or the other, the subject supposedly not being nursing or anyone else's concern except the client's, and lack of information. This rationale for noninvolvement is unacceptable elsewhere in health delivery, and it is just as unacceptable in delivering sexual health care. Sidestepping sexual issues leaves the health worker ignorant of an aspect of client functioning, a gap that may be a problem in later planning. If the client, for example, has prior sexual health concerns and no opportunity to deal with them, such concerns can become a hidden agenda in nurse–client interactions and block action on other issues. In short, hidden agendas in other areas of health functioning are empathetically sought out; sexual health deserves the same nonjudgmental care.

Constructive and nonjudgmental attitudes held by health workers are of inestimable benefit in counseling clients with **sexually transmitted diseases,** or **STDs.** Infections such as gonorrhea and herpes are seen in the perspective of being just that: diseases, not punishments for a particular behavior or choice of life-style.

STDs remain a constant public health problem. Antibiotic medication has been a mixed blessing: swift treatment on the one hand, complacency on the other. With some STDs affecting epidemic numbers, it is even more imperative that health workers include adequate information on these infections to those at risk. The objectives remain the same as in other health teaching: increase the patient's knowledge level, enabling them to make informed decisions, and provide secondary prevention to others exposed to infection, in this instance by contact tracing.

The discussion of STDs includes gonorrhea, herpes simplex (or herpes types 1 and 2), nongonococcal urethritis (otherwise called nonspecific urethritis), syphilis, vaginitis, and cervicitis.

# GONORRHEA

### *Characteristics of Infection and Clues to Diagnosis*

**Gonorrhea** is one of the oldest and best-established venereal diseases. It was hoped that antibiotics would bring an end to the disease, but gonorrhea has resisted control. Complacency related to quick antibiotic cure, ignorance about the infectious process of the disease, drug-resistant strains, and incomplete reporting and follow-up all contribute to persistent gonorrheal infection in communities. In the age group 15 to 35 years, gonorrhea incidence has increased steadily in recent years.

Gonorrhea is seen worldwide, with a greater prevalence in large cities and among male homosexuals with multiple partners. Gonorrhea appears to be one of the infectious diseases chronically underreported, so true incidence is difficult to obtain.

In males, gonorrhea causes a thick, yellow discharge that seeps from the urethra and is often most noticeable in the morning. The male patient will complain of burning and pain on urinating. Females may also complain of vaginitis or pain on urination, indicating urethritis. In women, cervicitis may be seen on examination and there may be some vaginal discharge, but the latter is often not as noticeable as it is in men. In either sex, the infection may be present at other "inoculation" sites such as the mouth, throat, or anus and rectum. It is possible for both men and women to be asymptomatic.

Treatment is usually sought because of discomfort and readily apparent symptoms, especially in males. In women, the symptoms are less obvious and the female patient may not be aware she is infected. If either patient ignores obvious signs and does not seek treatment, the symptoms disappear in one to two weeks, and the person may mistakenly think they are well. In women, untreated gonorrhea can travel up into the pelvis through the uterus and fallopian tubes. The fallopian tubes become infected (salpingitis), as does the pelvic peritoneum (pelvic peritonitis), producing an overall condition known as **pelvic inflammatory disease,** or **PID**. Untreated gonorrhea in men can lead to infection of the epididymis in the testicles (epididymitis) or the prostate gland in the pelvis (prostatitis) as the infection travels through the vas deferens. In both men and women, the inflammation and infection from untreated gonorrhea can lead to scarring of the vas deferens or fallopian tubes and subsequent sterility. Further late complications are a generalized illness with fever, malaise, and joint pains—an illness easily confused with others, such as influenza, unless a careful assessment has been made. The joint pains may persist, however, and develop into arthritis with acutely painful and swollen joints. These late complications appear more often in female than in male patients.

**Diagnosis** of gonorrhea is made by microscopic study of a smear of the discharge and by a culture of the discharge. On microscopic study, the smear is fixed and stained and the typical organism is seen, if it is present. Culturing the discharge will yield growth on the medium of typical organism colonies. Smear and culture are the diagnostic methods with gonorrhea, since blood serology is not readily available. In males, the discharge is usually apparent and readily checked; females may need repeated smears from the cervix as well as the urethra before the gonorrhea organism is demonstrated. In both sexes, the diagnosis of gonorrhea may be made more difficult by concurrent infection with other STDs, including syphilis. This leads to the practice of routinely doing blood serology for syphilis when checking for gonorrhea, so both diseases can be treated together if need be. Sometimes the gonorrheal discharge is complicated by another organism or infection that produces its own exudate; such a situation requires careful differentiation. One of the most common entities confusing a clear diagnosis of gonorrhea in males is a condition known as **nongonococcal urethritis (NGU),** or nonspecific urethritis. This condition produces a discharge and irritation, but the discharge does not demonstrate gonorrhea when seen under the microscope. In NGU, the discharge tends to be clearer than it is in gonorrhea, but it is more persistent. Since NGU is widespread among men, it needs to be carefully differentiated from the more serious true gonorrheal infection. The causative organism may be *Candida Albicans,* the herpes virus, *Trichomonas vaginalis,* or more frequently, *Chlamydia.* All urethritis needs careful diagnosis and treatment tailored to the cause.

Gonorrhea is also responsible for two other conditions: **ophthalmia neonatorum** in infants, in which the baby is exposed to the risk of blindness caused by gonorrhea present in the vagina at birth, and **gonococcal vulvovaginitis** in little girls, with vulval inflammation and vaginal discharge caused by contracting gonorrhea from someone else in the immediate household. Ophthalmia neonatorum is treated by instilling penicillin or silver nitrate drops into the newborn's eyes within a few minutes of birth, vulvovaginitis will run its course with recovery in a few weeks or months. The latter entity does, however, require follow-up with the family; the comments on contact tracing also apply here.

### Responsible Organism

The bacteria responsible for gonorrhea is the **gonococcus,** or **Neisseria gonorrhoeae**. *N. gonorrhoeae* is a diplococcus, or paired bacteria; under the microscope it resembles the two cut halves of an orange, with the rounded sides outside and the flattened sides next to each other. Gonorrheal diplococci need a warm, moist environment in order to grow, do not survive very long outside the body, and are particularly susceptible to drying conditions. Bacteriologists describe *N. gonorrhoeae* as a gram-negative intracellular diplococcus; this means the diplococci do not retain a dye solution (negate it) and, in order to be visualized on the slide, must be dyed with a second solution. This second solution is taken up by the organism, clearly outlining the typical paired bacteria with their flattened inside surfaces. The staining procedure takes only a few minutes and can yield a quick presumptive diagnosis. The discharge is also grown on a laboratory culture medium for 24 to 48 hours; if the bacterial colonies grown are *N. gonorrhoeae,* this confirms the diagnosis.

### Transmission of the Disease

Gonorrhea is passed from person to person by direct, intimate, sexual contact with infected mucous membranes of the vagina, penis, mouth, or anus and rectum. In gonococcal vulvovaginitis in little girls, the organism is transmitted by direct contact with the discharge from an infected adult in the home or by sexual contact with an infected adult.

### Treatment and Control

There is no immunity to gonorrhea, repeated infection is common, and anyone exposed is susceptible. Once exposed, the incubation period is usually short, with symptoms of dysuria (pain on urinating) and discharge appearing in two to four days. Men and women who do not realize they are infected or who ignore symptoms of infection are carriers of the disease and remain contagious until adequately treated.

Gonorrhea is treated with penicillin, given intramuscularly or orally, accompanied by a drug called probenecid, which acts as a type of adjuvant in helping to keep the penicillin level high in the patient's blood (see Chapter 3 for an explanation of the adjuvant effect). A vital aspect of treatment is the return visit to ascertain if the infection is eliminated; this is called the **test of cure** and, in gonorrhea, is done one week after the initial antibiotic therapy. The test of cure will also uncover any penicillin-resistant strain of gonococcus; that is, if treatment has been thorough and the organism is still present, a resistant strain is suspected. Strains of gonorrhea resistant to penicillin are becoming more frequent and are endemic in some countries (e.g., Vietnam and the Philippines). Travel to and from these countries must be taken into account when assessing clients for care. Other antibiotics, such as tetracycline or erythromycin, are used in treating resistant strains or if the patient is sensitive to penicillin.

Besides teaching about the test for cure, nurses should stress to patients that self-medication, such as passing around oral penicillin medication among friends, poses the risk of inadequately treated gonorrhea, which may go on to produce later symptoms. Secondhand drugs may also lead to resistant strains of the infection. Client teaching must further emphasize abstinence from sexual contact until treatment has produced a test of cure for the person initially seeking treatment as well as for their partners. Gonorrhea treatment can be complicated by the coexistence of other STDs, and the client must be made aware of the possibility of prolonged treatment to clear all infections effectively.

**Control** of gonorrhea involves educating the public about STDs, especially people in the late teen and young adult years, who are often sexually active. Antibiotics produce a swift cure, but they do not replace knowledge about gonorrhea and related infections. Antibiotics also do not replace the use of a condom, which helps prevent gonorrhea. Prompt case finding, diagnosis, and treatment also contribute to control and are better utilized by those knowing about gonorrhea. For example, if women realize that gonorrhea is frequently asymptomatic in their sex, they can be further encouraged to ask for a regular check if their relationships are frequent and they do not have a monogamous life-style.

**Contact tracing** is one of the fundamental aspects of gonorrhea control. The person initially seeking treatment has to assume responsibility for those who have been sexual partners and therefore have been exposed to the risk of infection. Without breaking confidentiality by naming the initial source of infection, contacts are telephoned or visited and asked to report for a checkup as contacts of an infectious disease, regardless of whether or not they have symptoms. If the contacts have exposed other persons, the ripple effect, or chain of exposure and possible infection, continues. Contact tracing is obviously more difficult as the number of partners increases, but all possible contacts must be asked to have a checkup and treatment if necessary until all tests are negative.

Difficulties in treating and controlling gonorrheal infections will be lessened if the nurse is able to establish a noncritical manner and approach the client with helpful information and conscientious treatment. Nurses have a significant role in educating clients about STDs in general and gonorrhea in particular, with the aim of raising the level of client health knowledge and functioning.


# HERPES SIMPLEX (HERPES TYPES 1 AND 2)

### *Characteristics of Infection and Clues to Diagnosis*

**Herpes infections** are not new. Over 25 centuries ago, Hippocrates coined the word herpes; today, more is understood about the diseases caused by this virus, but there is much more to learn.

The herpes virus is something of a conundrum. It is still not clearly understood why some people never suffer from a herpes lesion, some have an initial lesion that heals and never returns, and others have recurrent outbreaks of the lesions. It is known, however, that the virus has **two phases,** or stages, in those afflicted: **primary** or initial infection, which often becomes **recurrent** infection because of the ability of the virus to remain dormant in the body, sometimes for long periods of time.

**Primary or initial infection** with herpes results in the outbreak of small blisters one to two weeks after the first exposure to the virus. This is the classic "cold sore," but the initial contact can produce the lesion at other inoculation sites besides the mouth, for example, skin and mucous membrane surfaces such as the thighs and buttocks, the vagina, and the anus or penis. The blisters quickly rupture and enter a wet-ulcer state. Over the next several days, this is followed by drying and scabbing over. The lesions then heal, often leaving a little red scar that usually fades. During this primary infection, lesions are usually more widespread, last longer, and are more uncomfortable than when the disease is recurrent. Patients complain of burning and itching in the area and often have discomfort when urinating or having sexual intercourse. Fever and other signs of viral illness may be present (e.g., headache and muscle ache). This primary episode lasts about three weeks and varies widely in its clinical expression; some people are very ill, and others have relatively few symptoms. After the healing of the primary lesion, symptoms disappear, and the virus becomes **dormant,** or **latent,** in the body. About half the people who exhibited primary herpetic lesions will not have another outbreak. For the other half, however, the end of the latency period is signaled by another outbreak of the lesions. This return of infection is called **recurrent infection.** In this stage the lesions tend to be smaller and less painful, and they dry and heal over sooner. In other words, recurrent attacks are just like the initial episode but generally less severe. One of the difficult aspects of recurrent attacks of herpes is their unpredictability. Recurrences may occur once a lifetime, once a year, several times a year, or as frequently as three to four times a month. Recurrent herpes can be extremely unpleasant and trying to live with; it is reassuring to know that only a small percentage of people have frequent recurrences and that almost all of these people will have fewer recurrences after the first year or two of living with the infections.

Recurrent herpes lesions are often triggered by single or combined factors. It is helpful in counseling clients with herpes to assist them in delineating their own **trigger factors.** The triggers can include stress, sunlight, fever, menstruation, drugs, or sexual intercourse. In fact, there are no general rules for herpes infections; there are individual patterns and trigger factors in each person.

## NEONATAL HERPES

Because of their immature immune response system, newborns have little defense against herpes infection. The virus is not contracted in utero but is passed to the infant during birth if there are active vaginal lesions. There is a mortality rate of nearly 100% in neonates infected with herpes. After the age of 8 days, permanent damage, such as motor, intellectual, or emotional deficits, can result from herpes-induced encephalitis (Illis, 1972).

If labor is imminent and there are no active lesions present, a normal vaginal delivery may be performed. However, if there is a herpes outbreak, a Caesarean section will be done to prevent infection in the baby. In a woman with a history of herpes infections, the type of delivery is decided by careful observation of any lesion activity, along with virus culture. This combination will determine viral activity and, if it is quiescent, permit a safe vaginal delivery.

## HERPES INFECTIONS AND CERVICAL CANCER

A further threat to women is the association between herpes infections and cancer of the cervix. In general, there is a very low incidence of cervical cancer in the population. Women with herpes simplex infections are at slightly higher risk for developing cervical cancer.

Cervical cancers are slow growing and easy to treat if detected early. A Papanicolaou, or Pap, smear can quickly reveal uterine or cervical cancer at a stage in which it has produced no visible symptoms, has done no damage, and usually can be completely cured. Women who are subject to recurrent herpes infections should have a Pap smear done every six months. (The Pap smear is a screening test that detects changes in cervical tissue by microscopically examining the cells.) Advising clients to have this biannual Pap smear is an important item in the teaching related to herpes infections; the checkup also helps allay anxiety about the associated risk of possible cancer.

**Diagnosis** of herpes is usually done by clinical examination and a health history. Definitive diagnosis is done by laboratory culture of the virus.

### Responsible Organism

The herpes virus is one of a family of viruses that includes herpes zoster (chickenpox and shingles, Chapter 7), the Epstein-Barr (EB) virus (infectious mononucleosis, Chapter 9), and cytomegalovirus (responsible for congenital infant infection, but not a threat to adults). These four viruses are related because they all contain a large particle of DNA coated with a protein and protected by an envelope. In contrast, plant and animal cells contain both DNA and RNA in their cells; viruses contain only the DNA. (DNA and RNA stand for deoxy-ribonucleic acid and ribonucleic acid, respectively. They are called the building blocks in the body due to their reproduction in the chromosomes of plant and animal cells and their ability to pass on hereditary characteristics.) This viral family is related by structure, but it can be seen that the viruses cause nonrelated, or dissimilar, illnesses. In fact, immunity to one member of the family does not give immunity to another in the family, nor does infection with one make infection with another more likely.

Viruses are **intracellular parasites;** that is, they can only live and reproduce by entering a living cell in the body. Once inside the body cell, the virus takes over the productive machinery of the host cell and begins reproducing itself. As the virus proliferates, it will cause this first host cell to burst, releasing thousands of new offspring virus particles that spread freely to neighboring cells and infect them. Eventually, the body's immune defense systems halt the spread of the virus as antibodies develop. This antibody development explains the difference in the healing process between initial and recurrent attacks of herpes. In the first contact, there is no antibody present, so healing is longer and the symptoms are often more severe. In recurrent bouts, the disease still occurs, but it is less marked and shows faster healing of the lesions.

Herpes simplex viruses may be subdivided, on the basis of types, into **types 1 and 2,** with the number describing the virus, not the severity of the disease. In practice, however, the viruses are extremely similar and sometimes impossible to separate. Usually, oral infections are of type 1 and genital infections are type 2, but this is only about 80% true, meaning that 20% of the genital infections are mixed type 1 and 2 or solely type 1. Furthermore, as oral sexual contact becomes more prevalent in our society, these numbers will change. The location of the infection is of much greater significance than its type.

**Latency** or a **dormant period** is another characteristic of the family containing the herpes virus. During the primary infection, the virus comes in contact with the nerve endings supplying the area of infection. The virus finds its way into the nerve ending and travels up the nerve to the first available resting spot, the ganglion. These ganglia form a chain of "switching houses" down the length of the spinal cord and are an integral part of the electrical network of the nervous system. In herpes, the ganglion infected is the one supplying nerve endings for the area of infected skin. For example, a lesion on the lips or in the mouth travels to the trigeminal ganglion, while a genital lesion ends up in the sacral ganglion. In a process not yet understood, the virus becomes latent in the ganglia (i.e., it rests in the nerve cell and causes no symptoms). Meanwhile, the skin heals and the immune system destroys the virus in the skin.

**Recurrent disease** occurs when the virus stirs from its latency in the ganglion, travels back down the nerve ending it previously ascended, and causes new lesions to break out. The cycle of blister, ulcer, and healing repeats itself, but, with this recurrence, antibodies are now present to temper the severity of the outbreak. Antibodies, however, are extracellular: they can only kill the virus when it leaves the cell. Herpes, however, is a typical virus in its intracellular ability to spread from one cell to another by a sort of "tunneling" and without ever having to leave the host cell. This characteristic means that viruses are beyond the reach of many current treatment methods, such as antibiotics.

### Transmission of the Disease

Herpes simplex virus must come into contact with skin or mucous membrane in order to be infective. The virus does not travel in the air or live on toilet seats. In some tropical or poverty-stricken areas, however, the disease has infected over 90% of the population. In these areas, the virus may be transmitted by shared clothing combined with excess humidity or perspiration in the clothing and poor hygiene. In the United States and Canada, however, the virus is transmitted almost exclusively by sexual contact: oral herpes by kissing or other mouth-to-lesion contact, and genital herpes by intercourse.

A person is contagious from the time they get a warning sign (tingling or burning in the skin, itching, numbness in the leg), until the lesion has gone through all the stages (blister, vesicles, crusted ulcer). When the crust falls off and a layer of new skin is continuous over the sore, there is no longer any virus present. Residual erythema is not an active sore and will not infect someone else.

During sexual contact, there must be shedding of the virus from one partner in order to infect the other. However, a small percentage of people will shed the virus unknowingly. There are many reasons for this. If lesions are present on the cervix and nowhere else, they will be unseen and not felt because the cervix has no nerve endings to transmit feeling. The cervix, however, is usually not affected during recurrent disease, whereas it is commonly affected during primary disease. In addition, some people have lesions and do not know what they are or they may be very small and painless and go unnoticed. Although there is a small risk of spreading the disease by **asymptomatic shedding,** this disease is likely to be spread by contact with more than a minimum number of virus particles.

Thus persons who are prone to genital herepes infections must learn to recognize lesions and avoid sexual contact during periods of active infection.

### Treatment and Control

No therapy that has been tested to date has a significant effect on the herpes virus, including Herplex D, 2-deoxy-D-glucose, lysine, contraceptive foam, and even interferon. Presently, controlled clinical trials are under way to investigate the effectiveness of antiviral agents such as acyclovir (zovirax). Zovirax ointment should shorten the duration of genital herpes infections but not cure the disease.

**Palliative treatments** during an outbreak of genital herpes include

- Wearing loose-fitting clothing.
- Taking frequent warm soaks in a tub (sitz baths).
- Drying the lesions frequently with a blow dryer.
- Avoiding anything that keeps the area moist, such as ointments or creams.

These home treatments can bring some relief for the discomfort.

To help **control** the spread of this infection, it is important that persons suffering from an oral herpes simplex virus lesion take great care not to expose susceptible contacts to the virus. For example, visits by community health personnel to families with newborns and very young children must be curtailed if the nurse has a current herpes lesion. The infection can be controlled among family members by teaching principles of good personal hygiene. Hand washing should be thorough, and sharing articles such as towels and clothing avoided. Strict isolation of family members with active lesions is not indicated, but they should be made aware of the chain of infection and take steps to avoid "linking up." For example, hand washing is particularly important with children having herpes type 1 lesions, since younger children have more frequent hand and face contact. People who wear contact lenses should refrain from using saliva as a wetting agent and should wash their hands thoroughly before putting their lenses in (see Skin Conditions and Infections, Conjunctivitis, Chapter 13).

If a person is asymptomatic and does frequent self-examination to check for recurrent lesions, the risk of infecting a partner is probably very small. Permanent avoidance of sexual contact is not called for under any circumstance; however, intercourse must be avoided when active lesions are present.

In personal relationships, a policy of "informed consent" would likely be the best approach. This means a person is entitled to know about a history of herpes infections in their partner; that knowledge allows them to make an informed decision about their own actions.

Individual susceptibility and resistance to herpes is another of the puzzles surrounding this virus. Why do some people demonstrate active lesions while others never do? Why do some people have one initial outbreak and no other, while others have recurring attacks? It may be a factor in the virus, making it more virulent, or it may be some characteristic in the person's immune response system that determines susceptibility and resistance. Presently, four out of five people in the United States have been infected with herpes simplex type 1 virus, an incidence determined by large-scale antibody testing. Apparently, anyone ever infected with the virus harbors the organism for life; autopsy studies confirm recovery of the virus in four out of five people. One out of five people harbors the herpes simplex type 2 in their sacral ganglia, with the implied potential for developing genital herpes if the virus is activated or triggered.

Couples who are struggling with recurrent genital herpes infection need nonjudgmental support, help, and encouragement. The infection, with its recurrent and so far untreatable nature, is discouraging and often leads to depression or changes in the couples' interactions. Certainly, sexual activity must be avoided when a lesion is present, and, since the man and woman might have different recurring cycles of the virus, there may be great strain placed on a relationship. Sometimes the emotional state produced by trying to cope with herpes is in itself a causative factor.

Community health nurses are in an excellent position to offer constant support and up-to-date information to such couples. This support is often seen in the continuity of care the community nurse gives. The couple can become comfortable with the nurse through a series of visits or contacts such as prenatal classes, newborn visiting, or in clinics offering health services to the young adult population.

The noncritical acceptance of the nurse, accompanied by thorough and thoughtful health teaching about control, greatly increases the client's self-esteem.

# SYPHILIS

## *Characteristics of Infection and Clues to Diagnosis*

**Syphilis** is one of the oldest and most serious SDTs. Control of syphilis was heralded when antibiotic therapy became available, but the disease is far from controlled, let alone eliminated. Public ignorance of the disease, antbiotic-resistant strains of the causative organism, poor reporting on the part of the examiners, and inadequate follow-up to test for cure are all factors contributing to a constant index of infection in the population. In addition, syphilis incidence is increasing (especially among the age group 15 to 35 years who have grown up with the so-called antibiotic "wonder" drugs) and, in many instances, without the teaching related to the classic venereal diseases.

Syphilis is worldwide in distribution, with a higher incidence in males living in urban centers. The male homosexual group in large cities is particularly at risk, followed by heterosexuals with multiple sexual partners.

Syphilis passes through **three stages**—the primary, secondary, and third (tertiary or late) stages. The **first stage** is characterized by a primary lesion, or chancre, which is an ulcerated sore often seen on the external genitalia. The primary chancre can vary from about the size of a dime to considerably larger. It may be painless. Men usually see the chancre on the penis, but women may be unaware they have this initial lesion if it occurs inside the vagina and causes no symptoms. The chancre may also appear at other "inoculation" sites such as the mouth, throat, anus, or rectum. If unnoticed and untreated at this stage, antibodies develop and the chancre heals over. The site of the ulcer may resemble normal skin or the healed chancre may become a firm lump under the skin; in either instance, after the chancre disappears, syphilis rapidly passes into the second stage.

The **second stage** is the most highly contagious stage of syphilis and is characterized by a skin rash. This rash varies in appearance and distribution and can resemble measle-like bumps over the body, a small, discrete, bumpy rash confined to the extremities, or a single patch of discolored skin. The rash in second-stage syphilis is most often seen on the palms of the hands and soles of the feet—not areas where an examiner would normally expect to see a skin rash unless alerted by a careful history. The other symptoms of secondary syphilis are fever, anorexia, lymphadenopathy, general malaise, and perhaps alopecia (hair falling out in patches). Again, except for the alopecia, this group of symptoms can be easily mistaken for a much less serious illness (e.g., streptococcal infection or influenza) unless the health history was thorough. If still untreated, the second-stage symptoms disappear, and syphilis passes into the third stage.

In the **third stage** the syphilitic infection is characterized by dormancy. The infection can remain latent in the body for years, or permanently, if no treatment is given. Occasionally, there are spontaneous cures in the third stage, but, for about 30% of infected people who are not treated, the third stage causes severe damage. This damage results from the causative bacteria localizing in a vital organ, such as the heart, kidneys, or brain, with subsequent infection and tissue destruction. The outward signs of third-stage syphilitic damage include crippling arthritis, blindness, deafness, fatal heart disease, brain damage and insanity, destruction of tissue in the joints with collapse (e.g., nose cartilage is destroyed and the nose collapses), and the development of large, open sores on the body. Because of the dormancy factor, these symptoms may not show up for months or years into the third stage.

In any of the three stages of syphilis, adequate treatment and follow-up will arrest and cure the infection but will not reverse any existing organ damage. Adequate treatment includes checking for other, concurrent STDs; coexistence among these diseases is common.

Syphilis is also a grave threat to a developing fetus with **infection occurring through placental transfer.** In the early weeks of gestation, fetal immune response has not developed, so there is less likelihood of fetal loss. After the sixteenth week, however, antibody formation is present and syphilis intrauterine infection may cause spontaneous abortion or stillbirth. If the fetus survives, the infant may be born with congenital syphilis or succumb in the early neonatal period. Congenital syphilis in infants displays some of the same symptoms of second-stage syphilis in adults: rash formation, possible chancre formation in similar sites (mouth, anus, external genitalia), and a persistent stuffy and drippy nose (Anderson et al., 1979).

**Diagnosis** in all stages of syphilis is by blood serology and microscopic study of a smear from a suspect lesion. The blood tests used are the Venereal Disease Research Laboratory (VDRL) test, a screening test that will become positive five to six weeks after exposure, and the more specific Fluorescent-Treponemal Antibody (FTA-ABS) test, which uses a specific antibody-antigen reagent and will show positive results in three to four weeks. The microscopic study uses a smear of the chancre exudate and is done using a process called darkfield microscopy.

Darkfield examination involves lighting the slide in such a way that the organisms appear white against a dark background, making them easier to identify. Blood serology may not show positive results in infants under 6 months of age, so diagnosis of congenital syphilis is made by darkfield microscopy of a smear from a lesion.

### Responsible Organism

The causative bacteria in syphilis is the spirochete called **Treponema pallidum.** Spirochetes are so named because of their spiral, or corkscrew, appearance. The spirochete causing syphilis is called pallidum because it does not take up a bacteriological stain but remains pale. For this reason, darkfield microscopy became the technique used to visualize and study this bacteria microscopically.

T. pallidum needs a human host to survive and will not live long outside the body. It is destroyed by disinfectants and soap and by exposure to drying conditions. In order to study the viable organism, bacteriologists must use a "flash-freezing" technique to keep the spirochete alive for some time.

### Transmission of the Disease

Syphilis is passed from person to person by direct, intimate contact with a moist chancre, usually during sexual intercourse. The use of a condom may prevent some instances of infection by blocking contact with the chancre. Open primary lesions in other areas (anus, mouth, etc.) are equally highly contagious, as are any lesions present on an infant's skin. The first and second stages are the most communicable; in infected persons, secretions such as saliva and semen are also contagious. Syphilis may occasionally be transmitted through blood transfusion.

In **pregnancy,** the spirochete can cross the placental barrier and cause fetal damage, abortion, or infection after the sixteenth week of gestation.

### Treatment and Control

There is no immunity to syphilis. Having had an infection seems to give some resistance to the spirochete, but this resistance can be overwhelmed by a large, reinfecting exposure to the organism. Once exposed, the incubation period is a few days to about three months, but it is more often about three weeks.

Treatment consists of large doses of penicillin, given intramuscularly. If the patient is allergic to penicillin, erythromycin or tetracycline can be used. The large doses of antibiotic make the patient noninfectious within 24 hours, but treatment must be continued for up to one month while blood serology continues to be monitored.

It is extremely important that patients receiving therapy for syphilis and other STDs continue treatment until their blood serology indicates no further infection. This is called the **test of cure** and is vital in preventing further infection. The test of cure also helps to pinpoint an antibiotic-resistant strain of syphilis. For example, if the person has carried through with an adequate program of therapy and the supposedly final blood work still indicates the presence of *T. pallidum,* that person's particular infection may be resistant to the antibiotic used. In such instances, more laboratory study is done to determine what further medication is required to clear the infection.

Counseling patients also involves thorough **contact tracing.** This, in turn, implies that the person seeking treatment for syphilitic symptoms assumes responsibility for sexual partners exposed to the risk of the disease. When conscientiously reported and carried out, contact tracing is effective in primarily preventing new infection in those contacts named. Without naming the person who is the source of the infection, the contacts are telephoned or visited by nurses from a treatment facility, told they have been named as a contact of an infectious disease, and asked to report for a checkup. Because blood serology may take some weeks to become positive, contacts are monitored until the length of time for possible positive results (the incubation period) is over. Both the contacts and the person originally reporting for care must be encouraged to abstain from intercourse and other sexual practices until they know they are free of infection. One of the obstacles to thorough contact tracing is, obviously, the number of sexual partners named and the chances of someone being forgotten or missed. The other obstacle is transiency: calling a contact only to find they have moved to an unknown address. Every effort must be made to overcome these obstacles; a constructive, nonjudgmental approach on the nurse's part will benefit both patient and contacts.

**Control** of syphilis extends beyond contact tracing into health screening programs for premarital couples and pregnant women using the VDRL test. In many states, couples applying for marriage licences are required to have this test done. Routine prenatal testing, before the sixteenth week of gestation, will prevent possible abortion or congenital syphilis. Neither of these screening measures for syphilis control is foolproof because some women do not seek prenatal care until late in their pregnancy (VDRL should be done whenever they do come for care), and because some states and Canada do not subscribe to mandatory premarital VDRL screening.

The final element of control rests with public education with a twofold emphasis: teaching about syphilis, especially aiming at the 15 to 35-year-olds, and raising people's consciousness to assume responsibility for their own and their partner's health. It is hoped that teaching and assuming responsibility for oneself and others will help to prevent syphilis infections or, failing that, alert people to seek prompt diagnosis and treatment.

# VAGINITIS AND CERVICITIS

### *Characteristics of Infection and Clues to Diagnosis*

Vaginitis and cervicitis are widespread afflictions in women, and many suffer repeated attacks hampered by a lack of knowledge about causes and cures. Some infections of the vagina and cervix are sexually transmitted; others are not. Both types of infections, however, tend to cause the same symptoms and are **diagnosed** by the same methods: examination, smear, microscopic study, or all three. Because of these similarities, characteristics common to both types of infections will be discussed first, followed by brief notes on certain individual infections.

Vaginitis and cervicitis from any cause must be fully assessed and a thorough health history taken, noting the symptoms and onset and whether or not the woman is using an intrauterine device (IUD) as a contraceptive measure. Any vaginitis or cervicitis must be adequately treated in order to differentiate between infection in the vagina or cervix and possible difficulties with the IUD such as endometritis or salpingitis. With infections of the vagina and cervix, any or all of the following **symptoms** may be present.

- Vaginal discharge, abnormal in amount or quality and often with an offensive odor.
- Burning, irritation, and/or inflammation of the genital area, including labial edema.
- Pain and burning while urinating (dysuria).
- Vulval itching, sometimes intense.
- Pain with intercourse (dyspareunia).
- Nagging pain low in the back or abdomen.

When assessing infections of the vagina and cervix, the patient's partner or partners must also be seen and treated, if necessary, regardless of the initial cause of the infection. Dual treatment prevents vaginal and cervical infections from becoming cyclical, (i.e., each partner reinfecting the other). Combined treatment for both partners is a basic principle in the care of all genital infections; however, if clients are being treated for a nonsexually acquired infection, they may misinterpret this rationale. A careful explanation is required to prevent misunderstanding. The couple is usually advised to abstain from intercourse during the course of treatment (again, regardless of the cause of the vaginitis or cervicitis), and the woman is reminded to continue treatment throughout menstruation.

One of the difficulties in treating vaginal and cervical infections is the coexistence of other organisms, for example, gonorrhea and a vaginal yeast infection, or trichomonal plus monilial vaginal infection. Nursing assessment is of paramount importance in helping to differentiate the organisms and counsel patients receiving combined treatments.

Following treatment, the client couple is given a **test for cure;** again, this is a principle basic to the treatment of all genital infections. The test for cure determines the effectiveness of the treatment, ensures that there is no residual infection, and greatly relieves the client's anxiety.

**Nonsexually transmitted (or nonvenereal) vaginitis and cervicitis** result from a basic change in the acid-alkaline balance, or pH, in the vagina. At the time of ovulation in a woman's menstrual cycle, the ovaries begin releasing estrogen. Estrogen, in turn, stimulates the cervix to begin producing secretions; the secretions, however, are alkaline and, in addition, consist of cells that contain glucose. In order to maintain the **normal 4.0–5.0 acidic pH** of the vagina, certain organisms in the vaginal walls, called **Döderlein's bacilli,** convert the secretions by releasing weak lactic acid. The whole cyclical process keeps the vaginal environment in balance, and the cells are constantly renewing themselves. If this balance is altered and the pH shifts toward alkaline (7.5 and up, 7.0 being neutral) and the alkaline secretions are higher in glucose, the result is an environment in which organisms will proliferate. Some of the unbalancing factors are pregnancy, antibiotic therapy, oral contraceptives, stress and fatigue, poor nutritional status, another systemic infection such as a streptococcal illness, diabetes, poor perineal hygiene (cleaning toward the vagina instead of away from it), tight nylon underwear and clothing, and so-called feminine hygiene products, such as sprays and douches. Alone or in combination, these factors may account for an alkaline environment and predispose the vagina to infection with yeast or fungus, called *Monilia* or *C. albicans.*

**Sexually transmitted vaginitis and cervicitis** are also aided by an alkaline and glucose environment; these infections are **protozoan *(Trichomonas)*** and **bacterial *(Chlamydia* and *Hemophilus vaginalis)*** as the organism responsible for nonspecific vaginitis. Bacterial infections also include the STDs discussed in the rest of this chapter, but the distinguishing characteristic is invasiveness. In other words, the vaginal and cervical infections discussed here seldom, if ever, produce acute systemic illness in contrast to bacterial invasion by syphilis or gonorrhea. Each of the infections named will be discussed in order.

### Responsible Organisms

*Monilia,* or *C. albicans,* is a yeast (fungus) infection that thrives in a glucose-rich vaginal environment, so it is commonly seen in pregnancy when estrogen levels are higher, as an unpleasant side effect of oral contraceptives (which contain synthetic estrogen), after antibiotic therapy, and in women with diabetes. As the fungus proliferates, it often produces an irritating, lumpy, white vaginal discharge and vulval itching that may be intense. There may be edema and inflammation of the labia. Men can carry this yeast or fungus infection near the head of the penis, on the groove of the glans, or under the foreskin if they are uncircumcised. The fungus can produce a small sore on the end of the penis, and/or a fine, red rash over the perineal area. These latter signs must be thoroughly differentiated from syphilis, which is a far more serious infection.

## MONILIA

### Transmission of the Disease

Once monilia is established, regardless of the cause, it can be transmitted to the women's partner if she is sexually active. The incubation period varies from a few days to two weeks and is partly dependent on the recipient environment. If a man is carrying monilial infection, he can transmit it to his partner. If monilia is present in the vagina during delivery, the mother is likely to transmit it to her infant as **thrush.**

Monilia can be frustratingly recurrent, especially if the causative factors (e.g., diabetes or hormone administration) cannot be effectively eliminated or controlled. It is common for pregnant women to have recurrent bouts of this yeast infection; some women find monilia returning, to some degree, every month before menstruation. These recurrences are related to the pH changes in the vagina.

### Treatment and Control

This treatment involves both partners if the woman is sexually active. A fungicidal cream and/or vaginal suppository (nystatin) is usually effective if continued nonstop for 14 days and throughout menstruation. Occasionally, the monilial infection is also present in the intestine, and there is cross infection from the rectum to the vagina. In this situation, nystatin is taken in pill form, in combination with the topical vaginal preparation. The woman, or couple, may be advised to refrain from intercourse until treatment has resulted in a test for cure. Sometimes, even though the treatment has been carefully followed, the couple may be upset to find that the infection returns when intercourse is resumed. Such a recurrence is usually a result of intercourse smoothing out the folds in the vaginal walls and releasing some lingering yeast organisms. Seminal fluid is also alkaline, so the combination is enough to reactivate the infection in some instances. It is helpful to explain to the couple what is happening and suggest that the woman continue to use the fungicidal suppositories or cream after intercourse for an additional seven to 10 days. Her husband/partner could also wear a condom for this period to prevent renewing the cycle of infection.

Monilia in late pregnancy should be conscientiously treated to prevent neonatal thrush infection. If nystatin is not advisable, the pregnant woman can use mildly acidic douches, such as two tablespoons of white vinegar in a quart of water, twice a day. A test of cure should be done close to the delivery date, since infants exposed to, or developing thrush soon after birth, must be isolated in the nursery to prevent the spread of the infection to other newborns.

Monilia is not a serious infection, but it can be stubborn to treat and discouraging to live with. Women need to learn about the factors that can lead to an unbalancing of vaginal health and acidity; they can then make sensible decisions based on that knowledge. For example, it is surprising how few women keep an accurate record of their menstrual cycle. Keeping a record allows women to monitor any vaginal discharge and perhaps use a mild vinegar douche (two tablespoons of white vinegar in a quart of water) before their period if they suffer monilial recurrences at those times. Knowing about the glucose in the vaginal cells being shed will alert a woman to curtail extra sugars and carbohydrates, which metabolize into sugars, in order not to overload her body. In short, by doing some very specific teaching, nurses can increase a woman's awareness of overall health.

## TRICHOMONAS

***Trichomonas,*** or ***T. vaginalis,*** is more commonly known as "tric." This is a **protozoan** infection that is widespread in its distribution. Both men and women can have asymptomatic tric, and the protozoa can also be dormant in either sex for a considerable length of time (months to years). Women will seek treatment if vaginitis symptoms become pronounced, such as a profuse discharge and intense itching. On examination, the labia and perineum may be scarlet, and the discharge may have caused a fissure at the vaginal opening. Men seek treatment for symptoms of urethritis and may complain of tingling or burning while voiding.

### *Transmission of the Disease*

**Transmission** of *Trichomonas* is by sexual intercourse; it is common for partners to reinfect each other. Symptoms can develop anytime several days to 3 weeks after exposure to the protozoa, or the infection may be asymptomatic. In either instance, the protozoa can be seen by microscopic examination of a drop of fluid from the penis or vaginal discharge.

As in monilial infections, women with *Trichomonas* in their vagina can transmit the protozoa to their infant at birth, and men can harbor the protozoa under the foreskin if uncircumcised.

### Treatment and Control

**Treatment** of trichomonas involves both partners, and they must abstain from intercourse during treatment. The medication used is metronidazole (Flagyl), taken orally. It is effective for both sexes. Metronidazole is contraindicated in the first trimester of pregnancy; during that period, the woman is advised to use a vinegar douche instead (two tablespoons of white vinegar in a quart of water). A test of cure should be done close to the delivery date to prevent newborn infection. Besides being a risk to the fetus in the first trimester, metronidazole also has an adverse effect if combined with alcohol. In the latter case, the medication produces vomiting and gastrointestinal distress if there is alcohol present in the body at the same time, and patients must be alerted to this incompatibility.

As with other genital infections, the health teaching must stress concurrent treatment for both partners, and a **test of cure.** Couples should be warned that trichomonas may recur if treatment is interrupted. Even if the medication is properly taken by both, the couple may be distressed by a recurrence of symptoms on resuming intercourse. Again, as in monilial infections, the folds in the vaginal walls have flattened out during intercourse, releasing some protozoa. Treatment should be continued for an additional seven to 10 days, with the man advised to wear a condom to prevent the infection cycle starting up again. Couples need support and encouragement in coping with discouraging bouts of recurrent trichomonas.

### CHLAMYDIA

*Chlamydia,* or *C. trachomatis,* is a widespread bacterial infection producing many of the aforementioned vaginal symptoms. Many women, however, are asymptomatic until the infection has traveled higher into the reproductive tract to cause a low-grade pelvic inflammatory disease. The PID symptoms include abdominal pain and cramping, often becoming worse with each menstrual period. In men, chlamydia produces urethritis, and it is often the man seeking treatment with the woman being free of symptoms. Chlamydia frequently coexists with more serious genital infections such as gonorrhea.

Chlamydia causes ophthalmia neonatorum if present in the vagina during delivery, and in the neonate, causes a type of pneumonitis.

### Transmission of the Disease

**Transmission** of *Chlamydia* is by sexual intercourse, with reinfection between partners common. After exposure, incubation can be as brief as three days or as long as three weeks. The most frequent transmission pattern is from an asymptomatic woman to her partner, who then develops urethritis and, in turn, advises the woman to seek treatment.

### Treatment and Control

**Treatment** of *Chlamydia* in both sexes is with oral oxytetracycline. If the woman is pregnant, erythromycin should be used instead. Treatment may have to be combined if there are coexistent infections, and both partners should be examined and treated. A **test of cure** is also done following treatment; this is especially important if there has been concurrent infection with another organism.

As with other STDs, health teaching should stress that people who are sexually active with a variety of partners should have regular checkups to protect their own health and that of others.

### NONSPECIFIC VAGINITIS

**Nonspecific vaginitis** refers to an infection that does not demonstrate any of the preceding organisms while causing similar general symptoms. In addition to a vaginal discharge, the woman may also notice spotting or light bleeding that is not related to a menstrual period but results from the cervicitis present. Nonspecific vaginitis is often less severe than other vaginal and cervical infections, but it can be stubborn and resist treatment. The most common organism demonstrated in nonspecific vaginitis is *Hemophilus vaginalis,* which is a bacillus bacteria. *H. vaginalis* destroys the lactic acid produced by the Döderlein bacilli, and it is the absence of lactic acid and the presence of the typical rod-shaped bacillus bacteria that confirm the diagnosis.

### *Transmission of the Disease*

**Transmission** of nonspecific vaginitis is by sexual intercourse. The male partner develops symptoms of urethritis a few days after exposure; if hemophilus bacteria are the cause, they will be seen on a microscopic check of the urethral discharge.

### *Treatment and Control*

**Treatment** of nonspecific vaginitis includes both partners. If *H. vaginalis* has been diagnosed, treatment is with vaginal suppositories or cream containing tetracycline or a sulfa preparation. The male partner may be given an oral tetracycline preparation. Often *H. vaginalis* coexists with trichomonal or monilial infections particularly, since the acid vaginal environment has been temporarily destroyed by the hemophilus bacillus. The antibiotic or sulfa treatment is usually effective and may be combined with other medications if necessary. A **test of cure** is again advised for the woman or the couple.

## "HONEYMOON CYSTITIS"

This cystitis, possibly accompanied by urethritis, is a common complaint of newly married women who have not had frequent intercourse until their marriage (i.e., and honeymoon). Honeymoon cystitis is a result of the mechanical action of intercourse and not of bacterial activity. Frequency of intercourse, the thrusting of the penis against the urethral opening, and pressure on the vulva all combine to cause inflammation and tenderness of the sensitive, blood-rich tissues surrounding the urethral canal. In addition, the vaginal lubrication produced during sexual arousal may be scanty; this further increases the woman's discomfort. Honeymoon cystitis is usually treated conservatively after ensuring that there is no bacterial growth in the urine and bladder. Conservative measures include warm sitz baths (with no additives), a high intake of clear fluids, change of position during intercourse to relieve pressure on the vulva, and perhaps a short period of abstention until the inflamed tissues recover. Vaginal lubrication should be guaranteed during intercourse by adding a suitable lubricant if necessary. Petroleum jelly (Vaseline) is not a good lubricant; any of the contraceptive creams on the market, or K-Y surgical jelly, are recommended.

In summary, this chapter has dealt with STDs—some old, some new—that continue to create health problems in today's communities. Communicable disease of any origin breeds best in an environment of ignorance; this is especially true in diseases that involve the most intimate areas of human life and have, in the past, not been openly discussed. For their part, health workers cannot rely solely on the strength of antibiotic wonder drugs as a total cure; sexually transmitted disease is a health problem requiring honest and informative communication between the client and the nurse.

## ACKNOWLEDGMENTS

We acknowledge with thanks the review of material in this chapter by P. Lynne Buhler, R.N., B.Sc.N. Ms. Buhler is nurse clinician at the Medical Outpatient Clinic of the Acute Care Hospital, the University of British Columbia.

We also acknowledge the generous and expert contribution made to the discussion of herpes virus by Dr. Stephen L. Sacks, M.D., F.R.C.P.(C). Dr. Sacks is an associate professor in the Division of Infectious Diseases, Department of Medicine, Acute Care Hospital, University of British Columbia, Canada.

## STUDY QUESTIONS

1. The most prominent sign of gonorrheal infection, especially in males, is _____.
2. Culturing the discharge in gonorrheal infection is required as its symptoms can also be symptoms of _____.

3. A serious complication of untreated gonorrhea in women is
   _____.

4. Gonorrhea present in the vagina at birth can cause
   _____, in the neonate.

5. A basic principle in treating STDs is a _____,
   which determines the effectiveness of treatment.

6. Recurrent herpes is partly due to the herpes virus
   remaining latent in the _____.

7. A rash on the palms of the hands or soles of the feet
   should alert an examiner to the possibility of
   _____ stage syphilis.

8. Screening for syphilis is routinely done _____
   and _____.

9. Nonsexually transmitted vaginitis can result from a basic
   change in the _____ of the vagina.

10. Some factors that may predispose the vagina to yeast
    infections include _____, _____,
    _____, _____, _____,
    _____, _____, _____,
    _____, and _____.


# BIBLIOGRAPHY

Anderson, B. A., M. E. Camacho, and J. Stark. *Interruptions in Family Health During Pregnancy.* New York: McGraw-Hill, 1979. Ch. 5.

Austin, T. W., B. Lent, and F. L. Pattison. "Gonorrhea in Homosexual Men." *Canadian Medical Association Journal,* **119**(7), 731–732 (1978).

Benenson, A. S., Ed. *Control of Communicable Diseases in Man,* 12th ed. Washington, D.C.: The American Public Health Association, 1975.

Berkow, R., Ed. *The Merck Manual*, 13th ed. Rahway, N.J.: Merck Sharp and Dohme Research Laboratories, 1977.

Boston Women's Health Book Collective. *Our Bodies, Ourselves.* New York: Simon and Schuster, 1979. Ch. 9.

Cohen, S. "Patient Assessment: Examination of the Male Genitalia." *American Journal of Nursing,* **79**(4), 689–712 (1979).

Darrow, W. W. "Venereal Infections in Three Ethnic Groups in Sacramento." *American Journal of Public Health,* **66**(5), 446–450 (1976).

Fitzpatrick, J. E., N. D. Gramstad, and H. Tyler. "Primary Extragenital Cutaneous Gonorrhea." *Cutis,* **27**(5), 479–480 (1981).

Fouts, A. C., and S. J. Kraus. "Trichomonas Vaginalis: Re-evaluation of Its Clinical Presentation and Laboratory Diagnosis." *The Journal of Infectious Diseases,* **141**(2), 137–143 (1980).

Guinan, M. E., J. MacCalman, E. R. Kern, et al. "The Course of Untreated Recurrent Genital Herpes Simplex Infection in 27 Women." *The New England Journal of Medicine,* **304**(13), 759–763 (1981).

Hamilton, R. *The Herpes Book.* Los Angeles: J. P. Tarcher, 1980.

Hermann, K. L., and J. A. Stewart. "Diagnosis of Herpes Simplex Virus Type 1 and 2 Infections." In A. J. Nahmias, W. R. Dowdle, and R. F. Schinazi, Eds., *The Human Herpesviruses: An Interdisciplinary Perspective.* New York: Elsevier, 1981. Pp. 343–350.

Hobson, D., and K. K. Holmes, Eds. *Nongonococcal Urethritis and Related Infections.* Washington, D.C.: American Society for Microbiology, 1977.

Horos, C. V. *Vaginal Health.* Villanova, Pa.: Tobey, 1975.

Hume, J. C. "On Reports and Rapport in V. D. Control." *American Journal of Public Health,* **70**(9), 946–947 (1980).

Illis, L. S., and J. V. T. Gostling. *Herpes Simplex Encephalitis.* Bristol, England: Scientechnica, 1972.

Jaffe, H. W., D. T. Rice, R. Voight, et al. "Selective Mass Treatment in a Venereal Disease Control Program." *American Journal of Public Health,* **69**(11), 1181–1182 (1979).

Judson, F. N., and F. C. Wolf. "Re-screening for Gonorrhea: An Evaluation of Compliance Methods and Results." *American Journal of Public Health,* **69**(11), 1178–1180 (1979).

Kibrick, S. "Herpes Simplex Infection at Term." *Journal of the American Medical Association,* **243**(2), 157–160 (1980).

Kramer, M. A., S. O. Aral, and J. W. Curran. "Self-Reported Behavior Patterns of Patients Attending a Sexually Transmitted Disease Clinic." *American Journal of Public Health,* **70**(9), 997–1000 (1980).

Little, R. G., and M. Hartsfield. "Incidence of Asymptomatic Gonorrhea in Women." *Journal of Family Practice,* **7**(3), 597–599 (1978).

McCormack, W. M., R. J. Stumacher, K. Johnson, et al. "Clinical Spectrum of Gonococcal Infection in Women." *Lancet,* **1**(8023), 1182–1185 (1977).

McNab, W. L. "The Other Venereal Diseases: Herpes Simplex, Trichomoniasis and Candidiasis." *Journal of School Health,* **49**(2), 79–83 (1979).

Miller, B. F., and C. B. Keane. *Encyclopedia and Dictionary of Medicine, Nursing and Allied Health,* 2nd ed. Philadelphia: Saunders, 1978.

Moreschi, G. J., and F. A. Ennis. "Prevention of Herpes Simplex Virus Infections." In A. J. Nahmias, W. R. Dowdle, and R. F. Schinazi, Eds., *The Human Herpesviruses: An Interdisciplinary Perspective.* New York: Elsevier, 1981. Pp. 441–446.

Morris, W. S. "Epidemiology: The Community Nurse's Whodunnit." In S. Archer and R. Fleshman, Eds., *Community Health Nursing.* North Scituate, Mass.: Duxbury Press, 1975. Pp. 115–126.

Morton, W. E., H. B. Horton, and H. W. Baker. "Effects of Socioeconomic Status on Incidences of Three Sexually Transmitted Diseases." *Sexually Transmitted Diseases,* **6**(3), 206–210 (1979).

Nahmias, A. J., Z. M. Naib, and W. E. Josey. "Epidemiological Studies Relating Genital Herpetic Infection to Cervical Carcinoma." *Cancer Research,* **34**(5), 1111–1117 (1974).

Nahmias, A. J., J. Dannenbarger, C. Wickliffe, et al. "Clinical Aspects of Infection with Herpes Simplex Viruses 1 and 2." In A. J. Nahmias, W. R. Dowdle, and R. F. Schinazi, Eds., *The Human Herpesviruses: An Interdisciplinary Perspective.* New York: Elsevier, 1981. Pp. 3–9.

Noonan, A. S., and J. B. Adams. "Gonorrhea Screening in an Urban Hospital Family Planning Program." *American Journal of Public Health,* **64**(7), 700–704 (1974).

Odds, F. C. *Candida and Candidosis.* Leicester, England: Leicester University Press, 1979. Ch. 7.

Oill, P. A., and D. R. Mishell. "Symposium on Adolescent Gynecology and Endocrinology—Part III. Venereal Diseases in Adolescents and Contraception in Teenagers." *The Western Journal of Medicine,* **132**(1), 39–48 (1980).

Openshaw, H., T. Sekizawa, C. Wohlenberg, et al. "The Role of Immunity in Latency and Reactivation of Herpes Simplex Viruses." In A. J. Nahmias, W. R. Dowdle, and R. F. Schinazi, Eds., *The Human Herpesviruses: An Interdisciplinary Perspective.* New York: Elsevier, 1981. Pp. 289–296.

Overall, J. C. "Antiviral Chemotherapy of Oral and Genital Herpes Simplex Virus Infections." In A. J. Nahmias, W. R. Dowdle, and R. F. Schinazi, Eds., *The Human Herpesviruses: An Interdisciplinary Perspective.* New York: Elsevier, 1981. Pp. 447–465.

Parrish, J. A. *Dermatology and Skin Care.* New York: McGraw-Hill, 1975. Pp. 187–198.

Patterson, J. E. "Assessing the Quality of Vital Statistics." *American Journal of Public Health,* **70**(9), 944–945 (1980).

Rawls, W. E., and J. Campione-Piccardo. "Epidemiology of Herpes Simplex Virus Type 1 and 2 Infections." In A. J. Nahmias, W. R. Dowdle, and R. F. Schinazi, Eds., *The Human Herpesviruses: An Interdisciplinary Perspective.* New York: Elsevier, 1981. Pp. 137–152.

Rothenberg, R., D. C. Bross, and T. M. Vernon. "Reporting of Gonorrhea by Private Physicians: A Behavioral Study." *American Journal of Public Health,* **70**(9), 983–986 (1980).

Schachter, J., and C. R. Dawson. *Human Chlamydial Infections.* Littleton, Mass.: PSG Publishing, 1978., Ch. 7.

Schofield, C. B. S. *Sexually Transmitted Diseases,* 3rd ed. New York: Longman, 1979.

Shulman, J. A., and D. Schlossberg. *Handbook for Differential Diagnosis of Infectious Diseases.* New York: Appleton-Century-Crofts, 1980. Pp. 75, 218–219, 255.

Sumaya, C. V., J. Marx, and K. Ullis. "Genital Infections with Herpes Simplex Virus in a University Student Population." *Sexually Transmitted Diseases,* **7**(1), 16–19 (1980).

"Trichomoniasis and Other Sexually Transmitted Diseases." *Occupational Health Nursing,* **27**(8), 16–21 (1979).

Woods, N. F. *Human Sexuality in Health and Illness,* 2nd ed. St. Louis: C. V. Mosby, 1979. Pp. 107–118.

Yacenda, J. A. "Knowledge and Attitudes of College Students About Venereal Disease and Its Prevention." *Health Services Reports,* **89**(2), 170–176 (1974).

# 13

## Skin Conditions
## and Infections

When you have successfully completed this chapter, you will be able to:

1. Recognize conjunctivitis and impetigo infections in clients.
2. List the organisms that can be responsible for these communicable skin conditions.
3. Describe the methods of treatment and control used in combating these contagious skin problems.
4. Distinguish between communicable and noncommunicable skin conditions.
5. Describe nursing interventions for treatment of acne, eczema, and psoriasis.

Skin conditions often provoke an aversive effect in the viewer. In addition, there are noninfectious skin problems commonly confused with, or secondarily infected by, contagious conditions, complicating diagnosis and treatment. This chapter discusses two infections resulting from bacterial or viral contamination of the skin: conjunctivitis and the related sty, and impetigo. The additional noninfectious skin problems frequently encountered and often confused are eczema, psoriasis, and acne. These three conditions have an inherent risk of becoming communicable if infected with bacterial, viral, or fungal agents; for this reason they are included here. Information is also needed for taking health histories and making comparative clinical judgments.

# COMMUNICABLE SKIN CONDITIONS

## Conjunctivitis

### *Characteristics of Infection and Clues to Diagnosis*

**Conjunctivitis** is known as **pinkeye** because the most obvious sign is marked inflammation and injection, or reddening, of the conjunctiva. This inflammation is followed in a day or so by tearing and a purulent discharge that causes the eyelids to stick together overnight. The person complains of itching in the affected eye. Conjunctivitis is markedly contagious, the infection passing quickly to the unaffected eye and other people within two or three days.

Definitive clinical **diagnosis** is made by doing a culture and microscopic smear of the discharge. In practice, because of its rapid spread, conjunctivitis is usually treated after taking a history and carefully noting the signs and symptoms.

### *Responsible Organism*

Simple conjunctivitis can be caused by a number of bacteria such as staphylococci, streptococci, the Koch-Weeks bacillus, or pneumococci. A more serious form of conjunctivitis is caused by viruses such as the herpes virus.

### Transmission of the Disease

**Transmission** of conjunctivitis is by contact with the discharge or with contaminated clothing or articles.

### Treatment and Control

**Treatment and control** involves prompt exclusion of affected children from school or day-care centers, followed by the use of eyedrops or ointment containing an antibiotic. The medication should be instilled in both eyes to prevent the spread of infection from the initial eye and should be continued for a number of days.

Schoolchildren seem to be the most susceptible to this infection; the incidence decreases with age. Adults can contract conjunctivitis if they are in contact with the active disease. Patients and families should be reminded to launder towels, bed linen, and personal clothing thoroughly.

**Note:** Simple conjunctivitis responds quickly to treatment within two or three days. Patients or parents should be alerted that if such improvement is not seen, they must return to their doctor or clinic for a further differential diagnosis to be made. In some instances, the infecting organism in conjunctivitis is a more serious or difficult one to treat, such as the herpes virus, and delaying return may risk corneal ulceration or scarring.

*Styes.*    Styes are an infection in one of the eyelash follicles caused by one of a number of pus-producing bacteria. The stye resembles a miniature boil on the eyelid and, like a boil, it usually localizes, ruptures, and heals over. The discharge can infect other parts of the eye or body as a result of hand-to-eye contact. Styes are painful and they tend to recur. Occasional styes can be treated at home by warm compresses, paying particular attention to good skin hygiene and thorough hand washing. Recurring stye infections need to be followed up by doing a health history with the patient or with the parents, if it is a child with the infections. The health history will try to elicit factors in the person or the home environment that contribute to repeated bouts of styes, such as nutritional lags or gaps, especially in vitamin C, which helps maintain healthy mucosa, or the presence of skin boils in other family members. Another factor contributing to recurrent stye infections is **blepharitis,** an often chronic inflammation and scaliness of the margin of the eye lid. Since the skin is already irritated and often rubbed, especially by children, it is prone to becoming infected with bacteria such as streptococci and staphylococci carried on hands and nearby skin areas. Once clarified, the contributing factors as well as the infections can be reduced.

## Impetigo

### Characteristics of Infection and Clues to Diagnosis

**Impetigo** begins as a blister that breaks, oozes, and forms a thick, rough crust. The lesions most often occur on the chin, in the corners of the mouth, or at the edge of the nose. It can be a secondary infection to severe diaper rash. Impetigo must not be mistaken for a "cold sore," which is caused by the herpes virus. (This virus is discussed in Chapter 12.) Crusting face lesions in school-aged children are usually impetigo.

### Responsible Organism

Impetigo is most often caused by *Staphylococcus aureus* or streptococcus group A.

### Transmission of the Disease

Impetigo is transmitted by contact with the discharge from the weeping lesions or by staphylococcus residing in the nose. Children transmit the organism by frequent hand-to-face contact, as in nose picking or finger sucking. As a result, impetigo is especially common among younger children. Impetigo is not as flagrantly contagious as it was once thought to be; most lesions are autoinfected.

### Treatment and Control

Preventing the spread of impetigo involves prompt exclusion of people with the lesions until an appropriate antibiotic ointment is in use. Children should not be readmitted to group settings until the lesions are dry, since the organism is present as long as there is drainage. Early and adequate treatment prevents possible infection of other skin areas. Those having **repeated infections** should have a nasal swab taken and a culture done because some people carry *Staphylococcus aureus* in the nose and need more than local treatment. It is not clear why some people have repeated infections in spite of treatment and others have none. We do need to be aware that the very young and elderly are more susceptible to impetigo, as are those who are on steroid therapy or have some other chronic disease, such as diabetes.

**Primary prevention** can be accomplished with frequent, thorough hand washing, good skin hygiene, and minimal hand-to-face contact. Parents caring for their children's infections should be especially conscientious with hand washing.

# NONCOMMUNICABLE SKIN CONDITIONS

## Eczema

Eczema is a condition characterized by roughened, scaly, or flaky patches of skin. It is often of allergic origin. Depending on the sensitivity of the person affected, the skin patches can be fairly discrete or rather extensive: for instance, small eczematous patches on the cheeks or inner surfaces of elbows, to large inflamed areas involving most of the skin of the extremities and the torso. The affected skin can be dry and flaky, or vesicular, or weeping and broken, with fissure formation in the skin folds. It is often intensely itchy and made worse by stress, heat, cosmetics and soaps, and some fabrics, such as wool.

To parents coping with eczema in the family, it may seem as if the children were born with the condition, but a careful history, or knowledge of the children since infancy by the community health nurse, will rule this out. Eczema can develop, in fact, very early in infancy in a predisposed, hypersensitive child; to the parent, it seems as if "they have always had it." Children tend to outgrow extensive eczema; the skin becomes clearer as they get older. They may always have the tendency, however, to develop new patches of eczema when under stress or, if they are allergic to certain foods, a tendency that continues into adulthood. There may also be related allergies such as hay fever or asthma present in the same person.

The **treatment** of eczema may involve systemic desensitization (see Chapter 2) if the person has pronounced allergies. In some instances, children can be helped by conscientious monitoring and the removal from their diets of the offending food(s) that make the rash worse. Classic offenders are nuts, eggs, and some cereals. The affected skin can be treated by applying a topical ointment containing a steroid preparation to aid in reducing inflammation and promoting healing of the broken areas.

A risk with eczema in children, of course, is **secondary infection** from scratching, and, in infants, fecal contamination of the broken skin. Eczema sufferers of any age can contract a viral (e.g., herpes), fungal (e.g., thrush), or bacterial (e.g., staphylococcus) secondary infection, any of which may greatly exacerbate the condition. Needless to say, a person with eczema should never have a smallpox vaccination, nor should any member of the family if one person in the group has this condition (see Smallpox Vaccine, Chapter 6). Other antigens must be given with great care, taking into account the individual's allergic history. (Hypersensitivity, Chapter 2, and Screening the Vaccinee, Chapter 4).

## Psoriasis

Psoriasis is a conundrum with no definitive known cause and, seemingly, no effective treatment. Psoriasis can resemble patches of eczema or herpes zoster (shingles); the affected skin is dry and flaky or vesicular. As in eczema, the affected areas may be small and discrete or extensive and running into each other to cover large surfaces. Psoriasis seems to be made worse by stress. In some people, a period of high stress will result in an outbreak of psoriasis lesions, which spontaneously disappear as the stress level lowers. Most people with psoriasis, however, have had the condition for a considerable length of time and have tried many "cures." The use of topical steroids are often not as effective as they are in eczema; other ointments that are available vary in their ability to reduce the flaking and itching and promote healing.

Again, as in eczema, people with psoriasis are at risk of **secondary infection** with viral, fungal, or bacterial agents. Since psoriasis seems to affect adults more often than children, scratching the lesions is less a factor. Also, as in eczema, people with psoriasis should not be vaccinated with smallpox. Since there is not usually the hypersensitivity component to this condition, immunization may proceed after regular screening of the vaccinee (Chapter 4).

## Acne

Acne is too often regarded as simply an unpleasant adjunct to the teen years, and many young people do not receive proper care. There are differing types of acne, and a thorough differential diagnosis must be made by a competent dermatologist. Deep-seated acne of prolonged duration is more resistant to treatment than it is in the early stages and can cause permanent pitting and scarring of the skin. The latter is an unsightly and often preventable aftermath of inadequately treated acne. Nurses working in schools can be instrumental in initiating care and giving ongoing support and encouragement to the young person carrying out the treatment plan.

As with psoriasis and eczema, there would seem to be a stress factor in acne flare-ups. One of the stressors can be worry about another unsightly blotch! Hormone fluctuations during the teen years have also been implicated, but, interestingly, modern acne treatment is less concerned with the vagaries of the teen diet as a causative factor unless that diet is markedly biased toward high fats and sugars.

In common with psoriasis and eczema, persons with severe acne should not receive smallpox vaccination. To prevent further damage and infection to surrounding skin, the young people should keep their fingernails short and clean, avoid picking at the lesions, and observe overall scrupulous skin care, including frequent shampooing.

Each of these three noncommunicable skin conditions, eczema, psoriasis, and acne, has its own particular anguish for the sufferer. Treatments will change and hopefully improve as more is learned, but each needs painstaking care. Nurses are often in a position to support patients in a plan of care over a considerable length of time; this continuity may be one of the most valuable aspects of the treatment plan in skin conditions.

## STUDY QUESTIONS

1. Conjunctivitis is an inflammation of the _____, producing _____ and _____.
2. Because of the variety of causative agents in conjunctivitis, it is important to _____.
3. Health education as to the _____, _____, and _____ of conjunctivitis should be provided.

4. Impetigo is transmitted by _____ or
   _____.

5. Autoinfection can occur in children with impetigo by
   _____.

6. A risk associated with noncommunicable skin conditions is
   _____.

7. Allergy or hypersensitivity to certain substances is
   associated with outbreaks of _____.

8. A stress factor has been associated with outbreaks of
   _____ in adults.

9. A vaccination that should not be given to persons with
   eczema, psoriasis, or acne is _____.

10. The persistent nature of noncommunicable skin conditions
    requires _____, _____, and
    _____ from health care personnel.

# BIBLIOGRAPHY

Anthony, B. F., E. L. Kaplan, L. W. Wannamaker, et al. "The Dynamics of Streptococcal Infections in a Defined Population of Children: Serotypes Associated With Skin and Respiratory Infections." *American Journal of Epidemiology,* **104**(6), 652–666 (1976).

Benenson, A. S., Ed. *Control of Communicable Diseases in Man,* 12th ed. Washington, D.C.: American Public Health Association, 1975.

Champion, R. H. "Psoriasis and Its Treatment." *British Medical Journal,* **282**(6261), 343–346 (1981).

Chow, M. P., B. A. Durrand, M. N. Feldman, et al. *Handbook of Pediatric Primary Care.* New York: Wiley, 1979. Pp. 502–504.

Dajani, A. S., P. Ferrieri, and L. W. Wannamaker. "Natural History of Impetigo II. Etiologic Agents and Bacterial Infections." *The Journal of Clinical Investigation,* **51**(11), 2863–2871 (1972).

Dillon, H. C. "Impetigo Contagiosa: Suppurative and Non-Suppurative Complications." *American Journal of Diseases of Children,* **115**(5), 530–541 (1968).

Epstein, E. *Common Skin Disorders. A Manual for Physicians and Patients.* Oradell, N. J.: Medical Economics Company, 1979.

Farber, E. M., and A. J. Cox, Eds. *Psoriasis. Proceedings of the International Symposium, Stanford University, 1971.* Stanford, Calif.: Stanford University Press, 1971.

Ferrieri, P., A. S. Dajani, L. W. Wannamaker, et al. "Natural History of Impetigo. 1. Site Sequence of Acquisition and Familial Patterns of Spread of Cutaneous Streptococci." *The Journal of Clinical Investigation,* **51**(11), 2851–2862 (1972).

Frank, S. B., Ed. *Acne Update for the Practitioner.* New York: Yorke Medical Books, 1979.

Margolis, H. S., M. K. W. Lum, T. R. Bender, et al. "Acute Glomerulonephritis and Streptococcal Skin Lesions in Eskimo Children." *American Journal of Diseases of Children,* **134**(7), 681–685 (1980).

Mordhorst, C. H., S. P. Wang, and J.T. Grayston. "Childhood Trachoma in a Non-Endemic Area." *Journal of the American Medical Association,* **239**(17), 1765–1771 (1978).

Parrish, J. A. *Dermatology and Skin Care.* New York: McGraw-Hill, 1975. Pp. 112–117, 121–125, 150–154.

Quan, M. A., W. M. Rodney, and R. A. Strick. "Treatment of Acne Vulgaris." *The Journal of Family Practice,* **11**(7), 1041–1045 (1980).

# 14

---

# Streptococcal Infections

When you have successfully completed this chapter, you will be able to:

1. Describe the host response to infection with the streptococcus pyogenes in nonimmune persons.
2. Identify the signs and symptoms of four group A streptococcal infections.
3. Recognize the possible complications of streptococcal infections.
4. Explain how streptococcal infections are transmitted.
5. Instruct individuals and families in the treatment and follow-up of streptococcal infections.

Streptococci are a large and fascinating group of bacteria responsible for widespread and diverse illness. Because of the many varied clinical expressions of streptococcal disease, for practical purposes the discussion in this chapter covers those streptococcal infections most frequently seen in community health: sore or "strep" throat, tonsillitis, scarlet fever, and ear infections.

Whether the infection is mild or severe depends on the virulence of the particular streptococcal type and the overall health of the patient. In other words, not everyone exposed to streptococcal infections becomes ill. Such individual resistance to bacterial invasion is seen in many situations, but streptococcal illness gives particularly good witness to the phenomenon.

It is important to remember that streptococci can cause **secondary infection** in heart and kidney tissue even after apparently adequate treatment of the initial illness. Thus, a patient treated for tonsillitis, for example, may complain of urinary tract symptoms, or the person recovering from scarlet fever may develop symptoms of rheumatic fever. Acute glomerulonephritis is one example of kidney tissue involvement frequently showing up some weeks after a streptococcal throat infection and requiring prompt care. The person may have forgotten about the initial sore throat and not realize the relationship between the early and late infections. For this reason, it is vital to inquire carefully about any recent illness when meeting a patient with what could be streptococcal sequelae. Also, sequelae are particularly likely to occur in children and young adults who will not have developed as high a level of resistance to streptococcal infection.

## STREPTOCOCCAL EAR AND THROAT INFECTIONS

### *Characteristics of Infection and Clues to Diagnosis*

**Tonsillitis** and **otitis media** are responsible for much time lost from school and work. This pair of infections often occurs together or within a short time of each other; they provided the justification a generation ago for routine removal of tonsils and adenoids in young children. With streptococcal sore throat, the throat and tonsillar areas are red and inflamed, the neck glands are palpable and tender to pressure, and the person may have a low-grade fever and complain of feeling miserable. Conservative home remedies of rest, extra fluids, and antipyretic drugs, such as acetylsalicylic acid (ASA), will often ward off a full "strep" infection. However, if throat soreness worsens, pockets of whitish pus are seen on the tonsils, or an earache develops, the patient needs more rigorous treatment, such as antibiotic therapy.

If a sore throat responds to self-care and goes away in a few days, further infection is still a possibility because the streptococci travel through the eustachian tube to the middle ear. These infections require more than home care. Young children are particularly susceptible to middle ear infection, or otitis media, because of the alignment of the eustachian tube and the incomplete growth of the ear parts. Otitis media is painful because the streptococci cause fluid to build up in the middle ear behind the eardrum. As the pressure increases, the drum will bulge and, if left untreated, may rupture. This tearing brings relief from pain, but the drum heals with a thickened scar that can lead to **hearing impairment,** especially in the higher decibel range. In preantibiotic times, children often suffered recurrent ear infections with subsequent rupture and draining. Fortunately, this can now be avoided, but families may need reminding that otitis media can develop swiftly and treatment must be sought quickly. Children with such an infection who are too young to tell parents what hurts may be irritable and crying or may rub their ears. If the child has had a recent cold or sore throat, the parents should be alerted to seek adequate care for this possible secondary complication.

## Scarlet Fever

### Characteristics of Infection and Clues to Diagnosis

**Scarlet fever** is another expression of streptococcal infection beginning with a sore throat, fever and malaise, and, as it progresses, gastrointestinal upset. Before antibiotics, scarlet fever was a dreaded illness, especially in children. Nowadays it does not provoke the same reaction, but, if the patient or family seems to be overreacting to this diagnosis, check their understanding of scarlet fever and outline the current treatment. Occasionally, the name scarletina is heard or used; this term supposedly denoted a milder form of scarlet fever, but it is now out of date.

Scarlet fever has some characteristic clinical signs. One of the most prominent clues is the development of a fine, mistlike rash over the arms, torso, and legs. The second clue is that the face is very flushed but has no actual rash. Third, the skin around the mouth is pale, while the tongue is bright red. This latter sign is called strawberry tongue. The severity of the infection seen in scarlet fever is due to the ability of the streptococcus to produce a **toxin** against which the previously unexposed individual has developed no resistance, or immunity. Toxin production is further discussed in the next section.

As patients recover from scarlet fever, they may notice peeling skin (desquamation) on hands, feet, or other areas that had been covered with the rash. Second or repeat bouts of scarlet fever are rare because the person will have developed an immunity to the toxin produced.

Unfortunately, some people suffer recurrent sore throats and some children seem susceptible to repeated ear infections. In these instances, a full assessment of the patient's life-style may be indicated, with intervention planned, such as improved nutrition, to decrease their susceptibility to illness. In particular, everything possible must be done to prevent repeated ear infections and the risk of hearing impairment.

The postscript to streptococcal infection is teaching about possible **secondary sequelae.** Without alarming patients we can make it clear: they should return to their physician or clinic if any **cardiac or urinary tract symptoms** appear in the first few weeks following an acute streptococcal illness. Families need to know what symptoms to report; with acute **glomerulonephritis,** these are hematuria (blood in the urine), diminished output of urine, and puffiness (edema) in the face. There may also be a rise in blood pressure. These symptoms appear suddenly and are a result of inflammation of the kidney glomeruli and impaired filtration. Other reportable symptoms include chest pain and body joints that are hot, painful, and swollen.

### Responsible Organism

The streptococci are a large family of bacteria called by alphabet letters (A, B, D, G, etc.) and distinguishable only by serological study. The one responsible for the infections discussed here is **Streptococcus pyogenes,** a pus-producing strep. The S. pyogenes belong to group A streptococci; these are called hemolytic strep because of their ability to produce a **toxin** that "lyses," or destroys, the red blood cells. It is this toxin that produces the rash in scarlet fever; the previously unexposed person has not developed resistance or immunity to the toxin.

### Transmission of the Disease

Streptococcal sore throats (with or without tonsillitis or skin rash) are passed by person-to-person contact. Ear infections usually occur as a secondary complication of an initial streptococcal throat infection. Individuals may be healthy carriers of streptococci in their nose and throat and so infect others.

### Treatment and Control

Mild streptococcal infections are often self-limited, and an infected person may not seek care for this condition. However, if a close contact is known to have had strep, the throat should be cultured. This also applies to persons who exhibit a rash or have had rheumatic fever or kidney disease in the past. As a preventive measure, all persons under the age of 25 years, complaining of sore throat should have throat cultures. If the culture is positive for strep, treatment with antibiotics is begun. Either penicillin or erythromycin is used; both render the patient noncontagious in 24 hours. During this time, the patient should remain home from work or school. Patient teaching also stresses the importance of maintaining the full dosage of the antibiotic for the **total** number of days to prevent recurrence or sequelae.

Resistance and susceptibility to streptococcal infections is **type-specific.** This means that the person may be resistant to that particular invading streptococcus type, or it may be a type to which there is high susceptibility. It also means that an individual can be resistant to one type and fall ill from another, both from the streptococcal family. Then there are those who appear to possess high levels of resistance to streptococcal infections in general; those lucky souls seldom have a cold, let alone a severe "strep" throat!

Because of the widespread and diverse nature of streptococcal bacteria, **control** of infection extends beyond individual care to protection of food processing and handling. The purpose of extending control is to prevent "inoculation" of foods with streptococci. Milk and other foods contaminated by group A hemolytic streptococci can cause a miniepidemic of strep infection when ingested by susceptible people. Food preparation and serving must not be done by those suffering from sore throats, colds, or skin lesions. Milk should be pasteurized and all foods promptly refrigerated. These precautions pertain to homes as well as institutions; foods should be cleanly prepared and not left to stand at room temperature. A more detailed discussion of food contamination is found in Chapter 11.

Finally, the diverse *Streptococcus* family produces a multitude of illnesses not covered here, some of which are acute and serious. Health workers are encouraged to seek additional information in the extensive literature regarding streptococcal infections.

## STUDY QUESTIONS

1. The responsible organism in streptococcal sore throat is
   _____.

2. The sites of secondary infection after a streptococcal illness are _____ and _____ tissue.

3. The signs and symptoms of streptococcal sore throat include _____, _____, _____, and _____.

4. Children often suffer _____ as a result of streptococcal sore throat.

5. Circumoral pallor and the presence of strawberry tongue should alert the practitioner to _____.

6. Another clue to the diagnosis of this condition is a fine, mistlike rash on the _____, _____, and _____.

7. Symptoms of acute glomerulonephritis include _____, _____, _____, and _____.

8. Other reportable symptoms following an infection with group A hemolytic streptococcus are _____ and _____.

9. The presence of streptococcus in the nose and throat of an otherwise healthy individual is indicative of a _____ state.

10. An antibiotic regimen renders a patient noncontagious in _____ hours.

# BIBLIOGRAPHY

Baker, C. J. "Group B Streptococcal Infections." *Advances in Internal Medicine,* **25,** 475–501 (1980).

Benenson, A. S., Ed. *Control of Communicable Diseases in Man,* 12th ed. Washington, D.C.: American Public Health Association, 1975.

Breese, B. B., and C. B. Hall. *Beta Hemolytic Streptococcal Diseases.* Boston: Houghton Mifflin, 1978.

Gordis, L. "Effectiveness of Comprehensive-Care Programs in

Preventing Rheumatic Fever." *The New England Journal of Medicine,* **289**(7), 331–335 (1973).

Haverkorn, M. J., Ed. *Streptococcal Disease and the Community.* New York: Elsevier, 1974.

Kaplan, E. L. "Acute Rheumatic Fever." *Pediatric Clinics of North America,* **25**(4), 817–829 (1978).

Kaufman, A., D. Murray, L. Starita, et al. "Streptococcal Sore Throat Followup Program in a Hospital Clinic, New York City." *Public Health Reports,* **90**(4), 369–372 (1975).

Markowitz, M., and L. Gordis. *Rheumatic Fever.* Philadelphia: Saunders, 1972.

Marks, M. I., Ed. *Common Bacterial Infections in Infancy and Childhood.* Baltimore: University Park Press, 1979. Pp. 2, 83–85.

McCormick, I. B., and D. W. Fraser. "Disease Control Programs in the United States. Control of Streptococcal and Poststreptococcal Disease." *The Journal of the American Medical Association,* **239**(22), 2359–2361 (1978).

Molasanos, L. *Health Assessment.* St. Louis: C. V. Mosby, 1977. Ch. 8.

Rice, M. J., and E. Kaplan. "Rheumatic Fever in Minnesota II. Evaluation of Hospitalized Patients and Utilization of State Rheumatic Fever Registry." *American Journal of Public Health* **69**(8), 767–771 (1979).

Vickery, D. M., and J. F. Fries. *Take Care of Yourself, A Consumer's Guide to Medical Care.* Reading, Mass.: Addison-Wesley, 1976. Pp. 114–115.

Wannamaker, L. W. "Changes and Changing Concepts in the Biology of Group A Streptococci and in the Epidemiology of Streptococcal Infections." *Reviews of Infectious Diseases,* **1**(6), 967–973 (1979).

# 15

## Tuberculosis

When you have successfully completed this chapter, you will be able to:

1. Identify the factors that contribute to a person contracting tuberculosis.
2. Describe the transmission and progression of tuberculosis.
3. Discuss the diagnostic and screening tools used in tuberculosis case finding.
4. Explain the drug regimen and rationale for treatment of tuberculosis.
5. Demonstrate an understanding of the BCG vaccine in evaluating persons for tuberculin skin testing.

Tuberculosis is a venerable public health problem. The classic "galloping consumption" of past generations is now amenable to cure and prevention, but the number of new cases with a continuing index of infection in communities means that control and eradication are long-term objectives. Indeed, tuberculosis has a very persistent nature in humans. TB, as it is commonly called, is still prevalent in many parts of the world as well as being an infective risk for young people and large-city dwellers. Many health professionals, as well as the lay public, are mistaken in deeming TB conquered; in fact, proven management measures must be emphasized if prevention of infection is to be achieved. Many recent graduates in the health professions receive little or no tuberculosis education, an omission this chapter seeks to correct by discussing the proven measures for modern TB care.

### Characteristics of Infection and Clues to Diagnosis

TB infection enters the body by inhalation and prefers the locations in the respiratory tract that are best ventilated and supplied with oxygen. Since the initial defenses in the tracheobronchial tree are the mucous lining and the cilia, the organism has to overcome these in order to establish itself, grow, and produce infection. The only practical way the infection is acquired is by inhalation of droplets containing the organism; these droplets are expelled from someone with active, infectious TB. These invisible **droplet nuclei**, as they are called, remain suspended in the air, are carried by air currents, and inhaled. Indoors, the droplet nuclei remain infective for a very short period; outdoors, they present virtually no hazard because they are rapidly dispersed and are killed by ultraviolet light. (Before modern treatment, this latter knowledge was used as part of the traditional sunlight and fresh air treatment, along with prolonged rest for the lung tissue.)

In order to establish an **initial tubercular infection,** the droplet nuclei must penetrate the ciliary and mucous barri-

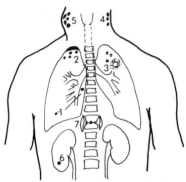

1. Healed initial infection in right lung
   (black indicates "healed" lesions)

2. Scars in upper lobe due to seeding
   (through blood stream) during early phase
   of infection.

3. Tuberculosis in left lung (with cavity) result
   of "waking up" of bacilli in scars.

4. Dormant (sleeping) infection in lymph nodes
   of neck.

5. Tuberculosis in lymph nodes of neck.

6. Dormant infection in kidney

7. Tuberculosis of spine (destroying parts of
   two bones and space between)

**Figure 15.1**   Sites most commonly affected by tuberculosis.

ers and implant in the alveoli or bronchioles or the lung surface, all of which are oxygen rich. The most **common implantation sites** (Fig. 15.1) are the alveoli in the lungs, especially the anterior surfaces, the lower lobes, and the apices. The initial infection in TB, then, consists of growth and proliferation of the organism at the implantation site in a susceptible person. This tiny, localized growth is called

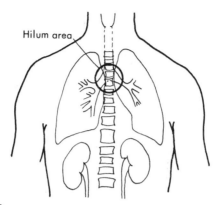

**Figure 15.2** Hilum or root area of the lung.

a **tubercle.** The early infection is often accompanied by enlargement of the lymph nodes in the **hilum,** or root area of the lung (Fig. 15.2). Body immune defense systems rally at this point and usually overthrow the invading organism. Occasionally, some organisms escape before the defense mechanisms swing into action, and the "escapees" may set up blood-borne infection foci in other areas of the body. However, the defense mechanisms generally are effective, and the initial site of implanted infection heals over, leaving a small deposit of calcium. These healed, primary lesions often escape diagnosis, except in higher-risk groups such as elderly, very young, or malnourished people. In these instances, and in others where the immune defense reaction fails, the tubercular infection progresses.

**Progressive tuberculosis** is an active disease process, with increasing areas of lung tissue involved in the infection; the causative organism is carried in the blood to other susceptible sites such as the kidneys. Progressive, untreated

TB carries the risk of **cavity formation:** the infection forms pockets, or cavities, in the lungs, which are filled with liquid containing large numbers of the organism. Progressive TB is the classic "galloping consumption" and, if untreated, is a pronounced contagion threat and can be fatal.

There is a **third category** of tubercular infection termed **latent, or dormant, TB.** In dormant TB, the initial infection site has healed, but the organism is still alive in the hilar lymph nodes and any other focus that may have been infected by the blood-borne, or escaping organisms. TB can remain dormant for a considerable length of time in the body, often **reactivating** under conditions of physiological stress, such as pregnancy or a systemic illness of some duration. The stages of tuberculosis are illustrated in Figure 15.3.

**Diagnosis** of TB is by a combination of clinical signs and symptoms, if any, tuberculin skin test (PPD or Mantoux), chest x-ray films, microscopic study of the sputum, and culture of sputum or gastric washings. In progressive, or very advanced late TB, the person will complain of weakness and fatigue, weight loss, periods of heavy perspiration at night while trying to sleep, and a chronic, productive cough that may be blood tinged. True hemoptysis, or the coughing up of frank blood, is a late sign of very advanced TB with cavity formation. The tuberculin skin test result will be suppressed giving a false negative, but the chest x-ray film will show extensive invasion of the lung tissue. Fortunately, the modern drug treatment for TB has made this stage an infrequent occurrence in community practice, but it must be differentiated from any possible malignancy of the lungs that can produce similar clinical symptoms.

People with initial, or early, infection will more than like-

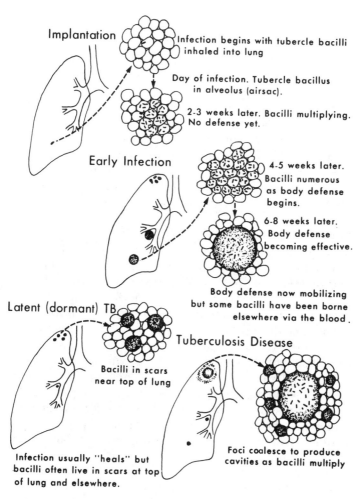

**Figure 15.3** Stages of tubercular infection.

**233**

ly have no demonstrable signs or symptoms. The best clue to diagnosis in these instances is the administration of a tuberculin skin test (a positive result indicates recent exposure and infection) or the less sensitive chest x-ray film. The latter will not pick up the very early infection, as does the skin test, but it will show any lung changes and healed lesions.

In either stage, but certainly in someone with signs of advanced TB, microscopic study of a smear of the sputum is done to aid in prompt diagnosis. The sputum smear is stained in such a way (see the following section on Responsible Organism) that the typical organism is clearly visible if present.

In groups of people at high risk for contracting TB, screening for early infection is a top priority in TB control programs. In addition, screening with the tuberculin skin test will also pick up those people with dormant, or latent, infection. The tuberculin skin test and follow-up rationale are discussed in detail under treatment and control.

The final diagnostic tool is a culture of the patient's sputum for the typical organism. This is done either by the patient submitting sputum samples for microscopic smear or by samples of gastric washings taken with the aid of a nasogastric tube. A culture of the organism requires eight weeks for results; the usual practice is to initiate treatment promptly if the skin test and chest x-ray show positive signs of tubercular infection. Sputum samples are submitted at the same time as this initial examination and diagnosis, and then treatment is begun. If future samples of sputum or gastric washings are needed, the patient must temporarily stop treatment before submitting the samples to the laboratory and restart treatment immediately after. If treatment is continued, it will depress the growth of the mycobacterium in the culture medium.

### Responsible Organism

Tuberculosis is caused by *Mycobacterium tuberculosis (M. tuberculosis)*, which is a rod-shaped, or bacillus, bacteria. There is a related mycobacterium, **M. bovis,** which causes tubercular infections in cattle and other animals. **Bovine tuberculosis** has ceased to be a threat in North America but continues to transmit disease from infected cattle to human handlers in areas where domestic cattle are not inspected and milk products are not pasteurized.

*M. tuberculosis* is described by bacteriologists as an acid-fast bacillus. This bacillus is peculiar in that it contains a great deal of waxlike material in its cells. This waxy material holds fast to a specific red dye in spite of a washing in both acid and alcohol (hence the name acid-fast). To make the red-stained organisms stand out on the slide, a contrasting blue dye is used, creating a microscopic scene of red organisms against a blue background.

Unfortunately, the property of acid-fastness is not unique to *M. tuberculosis,* but is shared by other organisms, called **atypical** mycobacteria. These atypical mycobacteria, as well as duplicating acid-fastness, further confuse clear diagnosis by triggering sensitivity to the tuberculin test. This means, however, that they act as a natural vaccine against any subsequent exposure to true TB infection by alerting an immune response. It is felt that while atypical mycobacteria do not always cause active disease, some seem to be pathogenic. The distribution of atypical mycobacterium is uneven; they are unknown in some areas and widespread in others, such as the tropics.

## Transmission of the Disease

In order to be infective, TB bacilli must be inhaled through the droplet nuclei, since the tubercle bacillus is nonmotile. The main source of infective droplets is the person with active, untreated TB who has sputum positive for the organism. Modern treatment methods quickly render such sputum negative. This means that in a population where TB is under control, as it is in the United States and Canada, a person is likely to contract the disease mainly as a result of occupational exposure (see Chapter 6, Occupations at Risk) or as a close or family contact of an undiscovered infection. In other countries where TB infection is highly endemic, there is a generalized increased risk of infection due to the undetected TB present in the population. TB is not highly contagious and, once exposed, the person is protected against repeat infections.

Mycobacterium tuberculosis requires the droplet mechanism for its transportation. In other words, a person is not likely to contract TB from handling articles such as books, furniture, or bed linen from a patient because the bacillus dries quickly when exposed to drying or heat and is not motile. Sunlight, or artificial ultraviolet light, will also kill the organism. Secretions that have dried and come to rest on surfaces such as floors are not a significant infection hazard for two reasons. First, the dried secretions do not readily break up and become airborne, and second, the particles that may become airborne are usually too large to penetrate into the lung; rather, they are trapped by the mucous layer or the cilia. Thorough hand washing is effective in removing any organisms possibly picked up from contact with the articles of patients.

Breaking the bacilliary chain of transmission from person to person involves **preventing contamination of the air** by the droplet nuclei from a person with positive sputum and eliminating any contamination that does occur. The prevention of air contamination is achieved by administration of antituberculosis drugs (chemotherapy) and by instructing the patient to cover the nose and mouth when coughing, sneezing, laughing, and so forth. The drug program reduces the cough and sputum in a few days; this is followed, in a few weeks, by a disappearance of bacilli from the sputum (i.e., negative sputum). This does not mean the disease is healed; it only means the patient is no longer excreting the bacillus through the sputum. Covering the nose and mouth with a clean tissue is effective in preventing the droplets from becoming airborne. The patient should be further taught to expectorate raised sputum into tissues, which are burned or flushed down the toilet.

Eliminating any contamination of the air that does occur is accomplished by good ventilation of rooms and the use of ultraviolet lamps. Both these measures are especially important in rooms used by patients before their drug program has had time to render their sputum negative.

It should be clear by now that the greatest contagion threat is the person with undetected TB with positive sputum. This is seldom encountered in today's community practice because of the TB "miracle" drugs, but safeguards cannot be dropped. One of the most effective safeguards is a consistent screening program for the detection of unknown cases, for example, chest x-ray films of all hospital admissions, or mobile chest x-ray films and tuberculin skin testing in highly endemic communities. Another effective safeguard is bacille calmette Guérin (BCG) vaccination for occupations at risk. These methods are discussed next.

### Treatment and Control

Effective drug treatment has revolutionized the care of TB in the last 40 years. Before the discovery of streptomycin, in the 1940s, tuberculosis care meant protracted periods of hospitalization that stressed bed rest, good nutrition, fresh air, and sunlight. It was also thought that a dry climate benefited the patient, so TB sanitoria were often built away from humid coastal locations. Families were often separated for months and even years while the ill family member was incarcerated in a "TB san." The social and economic consequences of the disease and its predrug treatment were enormous. Hospitalization is now required for only a very small percentage of active cases; hospitalization is determined by the activity of the TB, the client's life-style, and the ability to assume responsibility for the treatment plan.

The **drug regime** in TB is prolonged. While the medications quickly reduce the contagion threat by making the sputum negative, it requires lengthy periods of drug ingestion to heal the affected tissue completely. Patients may be required to take their medications for up to two years, or longer, depending on the response of their lungs as monitored by x-ray. Not only is the treatment prolonged, it must be **unbroken.** Full recovery depends on faithful adherence to the program with no interruptions in the taking of the drugs.

Tuberculosis drug therapy is based on culture and sensitivity of the patient's sputum or gastric washings. The usual initial treatment is a minimum of two drugs chosen for their effectiveness in killing the bacilli, thereby preventing drug resistance and relapse of the disease. Based on the laboratory culture, the drugs will be selected from several available choices and are a combination of two **first-choice,** or first-line drugs, or a first-plus a **second-choice drug.** Both lines of drugs, with related side effects and monitoring rationale, are outlined in Tables 15.1 and 15.2. A typical drug program, for example, might be isoniazid (INH) combined with para-amino-salicylic acid (PAS), or rifampin (RMP) with PAS or another second-line drug.

**Table 15.1** First-Line Drugs Used in Tuberculosis

| Drug | Side Effects | Monitoring |
|------|-------------|------------|
| Isoniazid (INH)[a] | Peripheral neuritis; hepatitis; hypersensitivity | Occasional serological testing (SGOT, SGPT). Pyridoxine may be given prophylactically, or as a treatment, for any neuritis |
| Ethambutol (EMB) | Optic neuritis, which reverses when drug discontinued; skin rash | Check red-green color discrimination and visual activity. Use with caution in patients with neural diseases or if eye testing not feasible |
| Rifampin (RMP) | Hepatitis; febrile reaction; rarely, purpura | Serological testing (SGOT, SGPT). Turns urine an orange color |
| Streptomycin (SM) | Eighth cranial nerve (auditory) damage; nephrotoxicity | Check auditory vestibular function (ringing in ears); audiograms. Serological testing (BUN and creatinine). Use with caution |

[a] Absolute contraindications to the use of INH prophylatically include previous hepatic injury due to INH, severe drug reaction, or presence of acute liver disease. Relative contraindications include chronic alcohol usage, pregnancy, patients on Dilantin, and patients who have chronic liver disease.

**Table 15.2**   Second-Line Drugs Used in Tuberculosis

| Drug | Side Effects | Monitoring |
|------|-------------|-----------|
| Viomycin | Eighth cranial (auditory) nerve damage; nephrotoxicity | As for streptomycin. Use with caution in older patients or those with renal disease |
| Capreomycin | As above | As above |
| Kanamycin | As above | As above |
| Para-amino salicylic acid (PAS) | Gastrointestinal upset, hypersensitivity, hepatotoxicity; elevated blood sodium | Serological testing (SGOT, SGPT). Frequently caused gastrointestinal upset |
| Ethionamide | As above, but with no sodium elevation | Serological testing (SGOT, SGPT). Divide dose to reduce gastrointestinal upset |
| Pyrazinamide (PZA) | Hyperuricomia; hepatotoxicity | Serological (SGOT, SGPT) and uric acid testing |
| Cycloserine | Psychosis; personality changes; skin rash | Difficult drug to use. Side effects may be masked by pyridoxine (see INH) |

**Monitoring** both the ingestion of the drugs and possible side effects is critical when the treatment is so lengthy. Community health nurses assume much of the responsibility for this follow-up by visiting the home and establishing a comfortable working relationship with the family. The follow-up extended to patients with tuberculosis includes teaching about the disease and its chemotherapy, assisting the patient and family with any laboratory requests such as sputum tests, and tracing contacts of the patient.

**Health teaching** with tuberculosis patients and their families should stress reassurance and support. A consistent explanation of the disease process will help families understand the necessity of adhering to the drug plan. Since most TB is now detected early, the person feels well and has usually had less interruption in their life from this disease than would be caused by a surgical operation. All of these factors can lead to a sense of false security, or even complacency, and the patient is tempted to discontinue treatment. Again, the nurse can use encouragement and give the patient opportunities to vent their frustration or anger at the drug regime or the disease. Families also must be reminded that the longer the infection has been present and the greater the lung involvement, the longer it will be before healing and restoration take place. The corollary of this teaching is that symptoms develop well after infection has become established, so the rapid disappearance of TB symptoms is only "the tip of the iceberg." A full course of treatment is their best insurance.

Health teaching also extends to primary prevention, if possible, for the contacts. In **tuberculosis contact tracing,** there is often a type of **priority rating for contacts,** with those closest to the source of infection as first priority, close, nonhousehold contacts as second priority, and other nonhousehold contacts as third priority. First- and second-priority contact must be reached, and, without compromising the patient's confidentiality, notified of their contact with TB and asked to report for either a tuberculin skin test or a chest x-ray. An effort must be made to do the same with third-priority contacts, but this is often difficult or impossible if such contacts are unknowingly exposed, have moved, or their location is unknown to the patient. Transient occupations are an example of a difficult contact situation. In short, prevention is carried out as far as feasible with as many contacts as possible.

Contacts are often kept under observation for a specific

time period, depending on their relationship to the original infection source. This surveillance may be repeat x-ray examination or tuberculin test in three months, or it may involve regular checkups for up to two years. One of the criteria for determining the procedure in protecting and following up contacts has to do with the results of, or changes in, the tuberculin skin test. Interpreting such changes is best done within the context of the tuberculin skin test in general; this is covered in the following discussion on screening programs for control of TB.

The **control** of TB infection uses a dual approach, first, to prevent disease developing in contacts of known cases of TB and the general population, particularly at-risk groups, and second, to discover the people with initial infections who do not exhibit clinical signs of the disease. Both of these control approaches rely heavily on the tuberculin skin test, otherwise known as the PPD or Mantoux, and an additional chest x-ray examination.

The **tuberculin skin test,** or **Mantoux,** is a preparation of five tuberculin units of a purified protein derivative of tubercle bacilli, hence the name PPD. The tuberculin material is injected between (intradermal or intracutaneous) the skin layers of the inner forearm. As the material is injected, a bump appears in the skin; this disappears in a few minutes. The test is read 48 to 72 hours later. In people who have not been infected with the TB bacillus, the injection site is indistinguishable 48 to 72 hours later. In those who have been infected, the sensitized lymphocytes gather at the site of the injection, causing a reddening and thickening of the skin. It is the thickening, or induration, that is the critical measurement. The erythema, or reddened area, can sometimes be quite extensive but should not distract the examiner. Induration is measured quickly and more accurately by holding the forearm up as close to the examiner's eye level as possible instead of looking down at the test site. If induration is present, it will be seen as a distinct "mounding" rising above the surrounding skin. The mounding can then be measured (in millimeters) by placing an appropriately calibrated ruler at a right angle to the swelling. Any induration should be recorded.

Health agencies, working in collaboration with tuberculosis control offices, establish a **minimum negative measurement,** below which no further follow-up is thought to be necessary. The negative reading is frequently 5 mm. A positive result is usually established at 10 mm. As this indicates, there is often a reading between 5 and 10 mm that is doubtful. If the doubtful reading is seen in a person who is a contact of a known TB infection, it should be interpreted as positive and futher follow-up (chest x-ray, repeat skin tests in an established pattern) instituted. If the doubtful reading is seen in someone from the population at large (i.e., a tuberculosis screening program), it is recorded, and may be repeated with a higher dose of tuberculin units if the person is from an at-risk group, such as a native Indian or a young schoolchild. The tuberculin skin test, repeated with a higher dose and often in the other forearm, will usually yield clearer results.

**Positive tuberculin reactors,** either contacts of known TB infections or screened from the population, are followed up with a diagnostic chest x-ray and possibly sputum or gastric washings. The procedure for following such reactors is, again, established by collaboration between health agencies and centers for respiratory disease control. Tuberculosis is a reportable communicable disease, so there is legislative involvement in its treatment and control. People with demonstrated TB found as a result of a positive tuberculin test will be started on antituberculosis drugs and followed up at regular intervals.

There are **specific contraindications to the tuberculin (PPD) test,** particularly with respect to the suppression of tuberculin reactivity. This suppression yields a false negative and occurs in instances of acute viral illness (e.g., rubeola, mumps, influenza), steroid therapy, pregnancy, and recent*(within four to six weeks) immunization with a live vaccine before tuberculin testing. If necessary, live vaccines may be given after the tuberculin test. Interestingly, people with very advanced TB give a false-negative tuberculin test. The tuberculin skin test should also not be given if the person has a skin condition such as scabies or extensive eczema (see Chapter 13).

The tuberculin skin test is a vital tool in diagnosing early TB infection in individual contacts, community groups, and those with early disease and no clinical symptoms. Because it is a health protection measure, especially in health- or food-related work, it is often an employment prerequisite. In all applications, the test is given and interpreted in the same manner, and this is an advantage. The test is quickly given and easily read. For nurses in schools, for example, mass screening of the children involves a minimum number of personnel and hours and is cost effective.

Tuberculin skin testing is also used to advantage to screen **populations at higher risk** for the disease. While theoretically anyone can develop TB, in addition to the close contacts of a known infection, other groups seem to be at higher risk. These include native Indians and Eskimos, newly arrived immigrants and refugees, people living in crowded inner-city areas, especially if nutrition is poor, and people with a history of lung problems (e.g., silicosis or emphysema) and/or inadequately treated "old" TB infection, perhaps before modern drug care. Screening programs for such groups are often done in a regular pattern, for example, tuberculin skin testing elementary schoolchildren every other year in the inner-city schools. The pattern of testing can be adapted to the ongoing test results: if the number of positive results is dwindling or increasing, the tuberculin testing program can be moved to another area or stepped up. The tuberculin test gives health workers a monitor on possible new cases of TB by providing a record of positive reactors in the community.

There is one other group that seems to be at increased risk of developing TB. This group consists of people who have had a tuberculin skin test convert from a negative, or doubtful, to a definite positive within the last one to two years. **Converters** are frequently, but not exclusively, contacts of a known case. The change from negative or doubtful to positive is a significant one for those who are contact converters and seems to carry with it an **increased incidence** of developing pulmonary changes typical of early tubercular infection. This increased risk needs to be spelled out to anyone who has had a skin test convert from a previous negative to a positive result, and especially to contact converters. The person who has converted will be further examined by a chest x-ray and may be asked to submit sputum or gastric washings for laboratory culture. Fortunately, the same drugs that are so effective in resolving TB infection are also effective in reducing the numbers of tuberculin converters who actually develop active disease. Thus people who have converted will be placed on a **prophylactic program** using INH or another first choice drug for one to two years. If it is sometimes difficult for patients with diagnosed TB disease to carry through with prolonged treatment, it is easy to imagine that patients might feel prophylactic chemotherapy is an unnecessary chore. Indeed, community health nurses must often summon persuasive teaching skills combined with consistent "keeping in touch" to convince families and patients of their need to continue medication. Nurses themselves must keep the essential issue of tuberculin converters—higher disease risk—clearly in mind when working with clients in this situation. As in treating active disease, a full course of the drug with no interruption is the person's best health insurance.

Public health protection from the undiagnosed and unsuspected TB infection is achieved essentially by screening programs using the tuberculin skin test and chest x-ray. There is, however, another measure used to give additional protection to people whose occupation exposes them to greater risk of TB infection (see also Chapter 6 for additional material on occupational disease risks). This category includes nurses, laboratory and related hospital staff, police officers, ambulance drivers, paramedics, prison personnel, and others whose work places them at higher risk than the general population. The **additional protection is BCG vaccine,** which denotes the bacillus of Calmette and Guérin, the two French bacteriologists who discovered the vaccine.

BCG is thought to give an 80% protection rate for a period of up to 15 years in people who are tuberculin skin test negative. In common with other vaccines, BCG is also thought to make less severe any TB infection that might be acquired in spite of vaccination. The administration procedure is in three steps. First, the person is given a tuberculin skin test which, of course, should be negative. Second, BCG vaccine is given within four weeks, but preferably within two weeks, after the skin test. Third, a post-BCG tuberculin skin test is given six to eight weeks after the vaccination, at which time the skin test should have converted to positive. This conversion situation is not the same as that in contact converters, even though the skin test result is the same. The BCG stimulates the body's immune system to produce antibodies to the injected bacillus, while the previously negative contact is indicating a possible exacerbation of actual disease. If the post-BCG skin test is still negative, it may be repeated with a higher-dose tuberculin unit (from 5 TU to 250 TU). If this second tuberculin remains negative, the BCG vaccination may be repeated in order to provide protection for the worker. Once the post-BCG skin test becomes positive, it remains so for an undetermined number of years, and these people should not have another skin test.

BCG vaccination is common in some countries where it is an integral part of TB control programs. Nurses need to assess whether families arriving from overseas have had the vaccination and make appropriate notation so they are not routinely skin tested, such as in the case of schoolchildren.

Nurses will probably not have to give BCG vaccination except in particular instances. In relation to other vaccines, there should be a three-to-four-week interval between BCG and other immunizations, and eight weeks between BCG and smallpox vaccination. BCG causes no serious side effects.

BCG vaccination, although safe and affording fairly high protection in tuberculin negative vaccinees, remains somewhat controversial. The difference of opinion has to do with the occurrence of atypical mycobacterial infections which, in some population groupings, create an immunity to TB infection and make those groupings tuberculin positive. For practical purposes, BCG is offered when contact with tuberculosis cannot be avoided in the community or family.

Modern TB care has done away with the family upheaval and disruption that once typified this disease. Community health nurses and other workers are now in a position to support and teach the whole family instead of have a loved and needed member absent in a hospital for many months. Historically, TB was a medical and family crisis; presently, it represents a situation in which community health personnel have another opportunity to build long-term, therapeutic relationships with the families they serve.

## STUDY QUESTIONS

1. Mycobacterium tuberculosis is described as an _____ bacillus because of its characteristic response to laboratory tests.

2. Five methods by which diagnosis of tuberculosis is made are _____, _____, _____, _____, and _____.

3. The prevention of air contamination by droplet nuclei is achieved through _____ and _____.

4. Four examples of first-line drugs used in the treatment of tuberculosis are _____, _____, _____, and _____.

5. A drug used in tuberculosis treatment that can cause eighth cranial nerve damage is _____.

6. Compliance with a medication regime in tuberculosis is complicated by _____.

7. In order of priority, the contacts that require follow-up in tuberculosis programs are _____, _____, and _____.

8. The control of TB infection through case finding and screening of contacts and at-risk groups relies heavily on _____.

9. The tuberculin skin test is read _____ to _____ hours after injection.

10. Groups at high risk for contracting TB can be protected by the use of _____.

## BIBLIOGRAPHY

Abeles, H. "Early Hospital Discharge of Tuberculosis Patients with Sputum Containing Acid-Fast Bacilli on Microscopic Examination." *American Review of Respiratory Disease,* **108**(4), 975–977 (1973).

Addington, W. W. "Patient Compliance: The Most Serious Remaining Problem in the Control of Tuberculosis in the United States." *Chest,* **76**(6), 741–743 (1979).

Addington, W. W. "The Side Effects and Interactions of Antituberculosis Drugs." *Chest,* **76**(6), 782–784 (1979).

American Thoracic Society, American Lung Association and Center for Disease Control. "Preventive Therapy for Tuberculous Infection." *American Review of Respiratory Disease,* **110**(3), 371–374 (1974).

American Thoracic Society and Center for Disease Control. "BCG Vaccines for Tuberculosis." *American Review of Respiratory Disease,* **112**(3), 478–480 (1975).

Bates, J. H. "Diagnosis of Tuberculosis." *Chest,* **76**(6), 757–763 (1979).

Benenson, A. S., Ed. *Control of Communicable Diseases in Man,* 12th ed. Washington, D.C.: American Public Health Association, 1975.

Comstock, G. W. "Advances Toward the Conquest of Tuberculosis." *Public Health Reports,* **95**(5), 444–450 (1980).

Dandoy, S., and K. Wiggins. "Current Status of General Hospital Use for Patients With Tuberculosis in the United States: An Update." *American Review of Respiratory Disease,* **110**(4), 442–445 (1974).

*Diagnostic Standards and Classification of Tuberculosis and Other Mycobacterial Diseases.* New York: American Lung Association, 1974.

Donaldson, J. C., and R. C. Elliott. "A Study of Co-positivity of Three Multi-puncture Techniques With Intradermal PPD Tuberculin. *American Review of Respiratory Disease,* **118**(4), 843–846 (1978).

Dudley, D. "Why Patients Don't Take Pills." *Chest,* **76**(6), 744–749 (1979).

Enarson, D. A., M. J. Ashley, S. Grzybowski, et al. "Non-Respiratory Tuberculosis in Canada." *American Journal of Epidemiology,* **112**(3), 341–351 (1980).

Fox, W. "The Chemotherapy of Pulmonary Tuberculosis: A Review." *Chest,* **76**(6), 785–796 (1979).

Glassroth, J., A. G. Robins, and D. E. Snider. "Tuberculosis in the 1980's." *The New England Journal of Medicine,* **302**(26), 1441–1450 (1980).

Grzybowski, S. "Strategy for Worldwide Control of Tuberculosis." *Chest,* **76**(6), 812–815 (1979).

Hershfield, E. S. "Tuberculosis in the World." *Chest,* **76**(6), 805–811 (1979).

Iseman, M. D. "Containment of Tuberculosis. Preventive Therapy With Isoniazid, and Contact Investigation." *Chest,* **76**(6), 801–804, (1979).

TUBERCULOSIS **251**

Kearns, T. J., and P. Russo, "The Control and Eradication of Tuberculosis." *New England Journal of Medicine,* **303**(14), 812–814 (1980).

Kopanoff, D. E., J. O. Kilburn, J. L. Glassroth, et al. "A Continuing Study of Tuberculosis Primary Drug Resistance in the United States: March, 1975 to November 1977." *American Review of Respiratory Disease,* **118**(4), 835–842 (1978).

Mitchison, D. A. "Basic Mechanisms of Chemotherapy." *Chest,* **76**(6), 771–781 (1979).

Nakielna, E. M., R. Cragg, and S. Grzybowski. "Lifelong Follow-up of Inactive Tuberculosis: Its Value and Limitations." *American Review of Respiratory Disease,* **112**(6), 765–772 (1975).

Pien, F. D., N. L. Michael, C. L. Ow, et al. "Primary Antituberculous Drug Resistance in Hawaii, 1957 to 1977." *American Review of Respiratory Disease,* **118**(4), 701–704 (1978).

Reichman, L. B. "Tuberculin Skin Testing. The State of the Art." Chest, **76**(6), 764–770 (1979).

Reichman, L. B., and R. O'Day. "Tuberculosis Infection in a Large Urban Population." *American Review of Respiratory Disease,* **117**(4), 705–712 (1978).

Rouillon, A. "Tuberculosis: A Model for Approaching Disease Control." *Chest,* **76**(6), 739–740 (1979).

Sbarbaro, J. A. "Compliance: Inducements and Enforcements." *Chest,* **76**(6), 750–756 (1979).

Standards Committee. *Canadian Tuberculosis Standards.* Ottawa: Canadian Lung Association, 1981.

Stead, W. W. "Control of Tuberculosis in Institutions." *Chest,* **76**(6), 797–800 (1979).

Steiner, P., M. Rao, M. S. Victoria, et al. "Persistently Negative Tuberculin Reactions." *American Journal of Diseases of Children,* **134**(8), 747–750 (1980).

Tizes, R., C. Hayden, and C. W. Tizes. "The Source of Notification in Tuberculosis." *American Journal of Public Health*, **64**(8), 809–811 (1974).

Wherrett, G. J. *The Miracle of the Empty Beds.* Toronto: University of Toronto Press, 1977.

# Answers to Study Questions

## Chapter 1

1. Any out of the following:
   Age
   Sex
   Ethnicity
   Genetic background
   Nutritional status
   Occupation
   Exposure to pathogens
2. Groups
3. Incidence
4. Prevalence
5. Immunizations, food and drug legislation, health education
6. Secondary
7. Rehabilitation
8. Contacts
9. Isolation or quarantine
10. Some examples are:
    Measles
    Hepatitis
    TB
    STDs
    Polio
    Rubella
    Streptococcal infections
    Any illness that has long been absent from a population

## Chapter 2

1. Kupffer cells
2. Digestion of the tissue
3. Neutrophils, monocytes
4. Interferon
5. Antigens
6. Humoral immunity
7. Specific
8. Adaptive
9. Boosters
10. Urticaria

## Chapter 3

1. Surveillance
2. Health teaching, immunization
3. Herd immunity
4. Never having seen an active case of measles, rubella, pertussis, or diphtheria, for example

5. Larger families
   Inadequate knowledge of vaccines
   Inadequate knowledge of U.S. and Canadian health programs
   Inadequate knowledge of severity of common communicable diseases
6. Law requiring inoculation before a child enters school
7. Public education
8. Adjuvant, depot
9. Risk factors, immune response
10. Placental passive

## Chapter 4

1. Convulsions or seizures
2. Contraindication
3. Immunization with a live vaccine, 30-
4. Does not
5. ASA or Tylenol
6. Hypersensitive
7. Histamine
8. Careful screening
   Preparation of syringe with adrenalin
   Counseling vacinees to wait 20 minutes postinjection
9. Intramuscularly, midthigh, deltoid
10. Hepatitis, abscess

## Chapter 5

1. 6
2. 10

3. Diphtheria
4. Sabin oral polio vaccine
5. The child maintains maternal antibodies
6. Increase herd immunity to lower the risk of fetal exposure for pregnant women
7. Three
8. 1:64
9. MMR, and DPT
10. Allergy to eggs, chicken feathers, and neomycin
    Untreated, active tuberculosis

## Chapter 6

1. Incubation period
2. Hepatitis, intestinal parasites
3. They are required to meet certain minimum standards for health status before entering a country (e.g., negative chest x-rays for tuberculosis)
4. Skin conditions such as psoriasis or eczema
   Pregnancy
5. Primary "take"
6. Adequate time (6 months) for vaccinations prior to any overseas travel
7. Six
8. Low-grade fever, malaise, local redness at the injection site
9. The elderly, especially persons with chronic

respiratory or cardiac conditions
10. Guillain-Barré

## Chapter 7

1. Winter, spring
2. Presence of all three stages of the skin eruptions
3. The torso
4. Shingles, herpes zoster
5. Person-to-person contact. Through contaminated articles
   Droplet or airborne secretions
6. Seven to 21
7. Crop of vesicles
8. Vesicles are dry
9. Stress
10. High-risk individuals, such as children with leukemia

## Chapter 8

1. Fecal-oral
2. Travelers
3. One, three
4. Four, six
5. Passive
6. Serum hepatitis
7. Anorexia, fatigue, abdominal pain, nausea, vomiting
8. Infected saliva or semen
9. Jaundice
10. HBsAg

## Chapter 9

1. Virulence of the virus, susceptibility of the exposed

person
2. Enlarged livers, enlarged spleens
3. Fever, lymphadenopathy, sore throat, malaise, and fatigue
4. PBD
5. Epstein-Barr
6. Mononuclear lymphocyte
7. Nose, throat, weeks
8. Older children, young adults
9. About two weeks
10. Is not

## Chapter 10

1. Regularly inspect school children and other groups
2. Insecticides
3. Griseofulvin
4. Contact with contaminated articles such as towels
5. *Sarcoptes scabiei,* direct contact
6. Itchy
7. Defecation
8. Vehicles
9. Avoiding foods and water where fecal contamination is possible
10. Toxoplasmosis

## Chapter 11

1. Salmonella
2. 12 to 36 hours
3. Fever, headache, abdominal cramps, diarrhea, and vomiting

4. Farmyard animals, especially poultry, domestic pets
5. Infection of raw meat
   Vectors such as insects, birds, vermin, or domestic pets
   Human carriers
6. Inadequately cooked, contaminated after cooking
7. Elderly, very young, or sick
8. Meat thermometer
9. Unpasteurized honey
10. Sudden occurrence of illness within a short period of time by persons who have consumed one or more foods in common

## Chapter 12

1. Burning and pain when urinating
2. Nongonococcal urethritis
3. Pelvic inflammatory disease (PID)
4. Ohthalmia neonatorum
5. Test for cure
6. Spinal ganglia
7. Second
8. Prenatally, premaritally
9. Acid-alkaline balance or pH
10. Pregnancy, antibiotic therapy, oral contraceptives, stress and fatigue, infection, poor nutrition, diabetes, poor hygiene, frequent douching, tight nylon underwear and clothing

## Chapter 13

1. Conjunctiva, redness, purulent drainage
2. Obtain a culture
3. Etiology, methods of contagion, treatment regimen (e.g., instillation of eyedrops)
4. Contact with staphylococci or streptococci in the nose
   Contact with the discharge from weeping lesions
5. Frequent hand-to-face contact
6. Secondary infection by pathogenic invaders
7. Eczema
8. Psoriasis
9. Smallpox
10. Support, encouragement, continuity

## Chapter 14

1. *Streptococcus pyogenes*
2. Heart, kidney
3. Red and inflamed throat and tonsils, swollen neck glands, low-grade fever, and general malaise
4. Middle ear infection or otitis media
5. Scarlet fever infection
6. Arms, torso, legs
7. Hematuria, low urine output, edema, increase in blood pressure
8. Chest pain, joint pain
9. Carrier
10. 24

## Chapter 15

1. Acid-fast
2. Clinical signs and symptoms (e.g., hemoptysis)
   Tuberculin skin test (PPD or Mantoux)
   Chest x-ray
   Microscopic study of the sputum
   Culture of sputum or gastric washings
3. Chemotherapy, covering the nose and mouth
4. INH, EMB, RMP, SM
5. Streptomycin (SM)
6. The length of time a person must continue to take medications
7. Close, household contacts
   Close, nonhousehold contacts
   Other nonhousehold contacts
8. The use of the tuberculin skin test and an additional chest x-ray
9. 48 to 72
10. BCG

# Index

Abortion, therapeutic, 80. *See also* Rubella

Abscess, *see* Immunization, sequelae of

Acne, 215-216
  primary prevention of, 216
  smallpox vaccination and, 216

Acute hypersensitivity, *see* Allergy, anaphylactic reactions

Adrenalin, as treatment for anaphylaxis, 62-63, 65

Allergy, 37-40, 103
  Allergen-reagin reaction, 39-40
  anaphylactic reactions, 37-38, 61-63
    emergency treatment of, 61-63
    mechanism of, 38
    types of, 61-63
  delayed reaction, 38-39, 63
  and immunization, 59
  types of, 37, 39-40
  *see also individual diseases*

Anaphylaxis, *see* Allergy, anaphylactic reactions

Antibodies, 22
  allergy, and production of, 38
  blocking of antigen toxicity and, 26
  complementarity of antigen-antibody sites, 25-26
  complement system and, 26-28
  formation of, 23, 24
  hepatitis B serum (HBsAB), 124-127
  Paul-Bunnell-Davidsohn, 132
  placental barrier and, 49-50, 72
  reactive site of, 26
  reagin, 39
  sensitizing, 39
  specificity of, 24, 26
  structure of, 25
  titer of, 48-50
  vaccination and production of, 32-33, 48
  valences of, 26

Antibody response, in infants, 8, 49-50

Antigen-antibody complex, 25-28
  precipitation of, 26
  susceptibility to phagocytosis of, 26

Antigens, 21
  administration of, 65-66
  of attenuated organisms, 32
  combined, 71-83

of hepatitis B, specific surface
(HBsAg), 124-127
safe handling of, 65
swamping effect of, 36
types of, 48
Antihistaminic drugs, 40, 62-63
Ascariasis, 148-151
organism responsible for, characteristics of, 149, 150
preventive measures for control
of, 150
signs and symptoms of, 149
transmission of, 149
treatment of, 150-151
Asphyxia, 62
Asthma, 40, 61-62, 214
Autoimmune diseases, 36-37

Bacteria, 28
agglutination of, 28
gram-negative, 160, 172
lysis of, 28
Bacterial disease: acute humoral-
antibody mechanism and,
31
slow developing cellular immunity and, 31
B-cells, 34-35
Body fluids, cleansing of, 17, 18
reticuloendothelial cells and, 17
white blood cells and, 18
Botulism, paralytic toxin of, 21,
32, 163
Brucellosis, 31
Burkitt's Lymphoma, 132-133
Bursa of Fabricius, 34

Candida albicans, 171, 194-197.
See also Monilia; Urethritis,

nongonococcal
Cellular immunity, see Immunity,
adaptive
Cellutoxins, 31
Cervicitis, 191-202
health education and, 192-193
health history and, 191
intrauterine device (IUD) and,
191-192
nonsexually transmitted, 193,
194-197
acid-alkaline balance of
vagina and, 193-194
Döderlein's bacilli and, 193
estrogen release and, 193-194
sexually transmitted, 194, 197-
202
symptoms of, 192
Chickenpox, 113-116
diagnostic clues, 114
immunity to, 116
signs and symptoms of, 114
transmission of, 114-115
treatment and control of, 115-
116
virus responsible for, 115, 178,
179
Chlamydia, 171, 198-200
health education and, 199-200
incubation period of, 199
opthalmia neonatorum and, 199
pneumonitis in newborn and,
199
symptoms of, 171, 199
transmission of, 199
treatment and control of, 199-
200
and test of cure, 199
Chlamydia tracomatis, 171, 198-200

Cholera, 90, 104
*Clostridium botulinum*, 163. *See also* Salmonella, epidemiological measures in controlling
Community health agencies:
  collection of information by, 9
  legislative actions and, 10-11
Complement complex, 26-28
  agglutination of bacteria and, 28
  composition of, 26
  lysis of bacteria and, 28
  mechanism of action of, 27
Conjunctivitis, 209-211
  bacteria and virus responsible for, 209-210
  control of, 210
  diagnosis of, 209
  health history and, 290, 211
  signs and symptoms of, 209
  styes, 210-211
    blepharitis and, 211
    recurrence of, 211
  transmission of, 210
  treatment of, 210

Damaged tissues: substances released by, 18
  "walling off" from surrounding area of, 18
Dane particle, *see* Hepatitis, B, virus responsible for
Dermatophytes, *see* Ringworm
Diptheria, 45, 70, 72-76, 89, 92, 101, 104
  vaccination, 73-74, 104
    reaction to, 75-76
    Schick test and, 73-74, 92
    specific contraindication

for, 76
  vaccine, 72-74, 89, 92
    antigenic strengths of, 72, 74

Eczema, 61, 95, 213-214
  allergy and, 213-214
  immunization and, 214
  prevention of, 213
  secondary infection, risk of, 214
  signs of, 213
  treatment of, 214
Encephalopathy, 63
Enterobiasis, 146-148
  organism responsible for, 147
  symptoms of, 146-147
  transmission of, 147-148
  treatment and control of, 148
Enzymes, digestive, 19, 20, 26, 28, 31, 38, 39
Epidemiological measurements, 4-5
  incidence rate and, 5
  vital statistics and, 5
Epidemiological methods, 44
  in eradication and control of communicable disease, 44
Epidemiology, 3-4
  definition of, 4
Epididymitis, *see* Gonorrhea, complications of
Epilepsy, 59
Epinephrine hydrochloride, *see* Adrenalin, as treatment for anaphylaxis
Epstein-Barr virus (EB), *see* Mononucleosis, infectious
Erythromycine, 173, 189, 199, 224

Estrogen, 193-194

Fibroblasts, origin of, 19
Flagyl, *see* Metronidazole
Fluorescent-treponemal antibody
          (FTA-ABS) test, *see*
          Syphilis, diagnostic tests
          for
Food poisoning, bacterial, *see*
          Salmonella

Gastrointestinal tract, lymphoid
          tissue of, 22, 34
German measles, *see* Rubella
*Giardia lamblia,* 151. *See also*
          Giardiasis
Giardiasis, 151-152
  organism responsible for, 151
  symptoms of, 151
  transmission of, 151-152
  travel and, 151-152
  treatment and control of, 152
Glomerulonephritis, acute, as
          secondary infection, 37,
          220, 223
  symptoms of, 223
Gonorrhea, 169-175
  complications of, 170
  control of, 174-175
  diagnosis, 170-172
  diagnostic methods, 171-172
  health teaching and, 174-175
  incidence of, 169
  incubation period of, 173
  "inoculation" sites, 170
  opthalmia neonatorum and,
          171, 172
    treatment of, 172
  organism responsible for,

        172, 173
    penicillin-resistant strains, 173
  reporting on, 169
  signs and symptoms of, 169-172,
          173
  transmission of, 172-173
  treatment of, 173
    and test of cure, 173
  vulvovaginitis and, 171, 173
Griseofulvin, 142
Guillaine-Barre syndrome, *see*
          Vaccine, influenza

Hay fever, 39-40, 61, 213
Health agencies, public, 45, 64,
          78, 91-92, 93, 158, 168,
          174-175, 243-244
  basic vaccine supply and, 74
  chronic illness immunization
          and, 105
  contact tracing in sexually trans-
          mitted diseases and, 174-
          175, 190
  small-pox vaccination for travel
          and, 95
  travel information on vaccina-
          tion and, 93
  tuberculosis control and, 243-
          244
Health education, 45-50, 64, 75,
          97, 101, 168-169, 173-
          174, 178, 183, 190-191,
          192
  for travelers, 97-101. *See also*
          Gonorrhea; Hepatitis;
          Malaria; Parasites, intesti-
          nal; *individual diseases*
Health program, 44-45
Health workers, *see* Health

agencies, public; Nurse, role in community health
*Hemophilis vaginalis. See* Vaginitis, nonspecific
Hepatitis, 66, 90-91, 97, 119-127
  A, 102, 120-123
    acute, 120-121
    immunity to, 121, 123
    incubation period of, 122
    diagnosis of, 121
    prodromal period of, 122
    signs and symptoms of, 120-121
    subclinical case of, 120
    transmission of, 122
    treatment and control of, 123
    virus responsible for, 122
  B, 101, 102, 120, 123-127
    chronic infection and, 124, 127
    diagnosis of, 124-125
    health teaching and, 126-127
    immunity to, 126
    liver malignancy and, 127
    prodromal phase of, 124
    serological test for, 124, 127
    symptoms of, 123-124
    transmission of, 125-126
    treatment and control of, 126-128
    virus responsible for, 125
  non-A non-B, 120
  as occupational risk disease, 66, 101-102, 119, 125-126
  screening of refugees for, 90-91
Herpes simplex (types 1 and 2), 132, 171, 175-184
  cervical cancer and, 178
    Papanicolaou (PAP) smear as

diagnostic test for, 178
  diagnosis of, 178
  epidemiological measures to control outbreak of, 183-184
  health teaching and, 178, 182-184
  immunity to, 180
  incidence of, 181, 184
  neonatal, 177
    rate of mortality of newborns and, 177
  as primary infection, 175-176
    symptoms of, 176
  as recurrent infection, 175-177, 180
    trigger factors and, 177
  transmission of, 181-182
  treatment of, 182
  virus responsible for, 175-184
    latency of, 176
    susceptibility of and resistance to, 183-184
Herpes zoster. *See* Chickenpox
Histamine, 18, 38, 39, 61-62
  effects of, 38, 39
"Honeymoon cystitis," 201
  treatment of, 201

Immune serum globulin (ISG), 66, 90, 116, 123
  chickenpox, prevention of, 116
  hepatitis, prevention of, 123
Immunity, 19-37
  active, 33, 35
  adaptive, 20-37
    cellular, 22, 29-31, 34-35
      impairment of, 35
      persistence of, 31

thymic lymphocytes (T-cells) in, 34-35
transplanted organs, rejection of and, 35
type of disease and, 31
humoral, 22, 24-29, 34-35
bursal lymphocytes (B-cells) in, 34-35
role of lymphocytes and lymph nodes in, 21-22
sensitivity of antigen in, 36
tolerance of, 29, 31, 36
type of disease and, 29, 31
vaccination and, 32, 48
antibody titer and, 48, 49
definition of, 19
herd, 45, 78, 104, 105
in infants, 49-50, 72-73
innate, 19-20
factors of, 20
passive, 34, 49-50, 123
placental barrier and, 49-50
side effects of, 37-40
Immunization: in Canada, 46, 77
chronic illness and, 105-106
complacency and, 45-47
of immigrants, 91-92
levels of, 44-47
national, 46
occupational disease risks and, 101-102, 123, 125. See also Hepatitis; Tuberculosis, bacille Calmette-Guerin (BCG) vaccination against; Vaccine, typhoid
overseas travel and, 93-101, 104-105, 122-123
health teaching for, 93, 97-101

public health agency information regarding, 93, 100
requirements and recommendations for entry into country, 94-97
pregnancy and, 60, 104-105
programs, 44-45, 47, 57, 60, 70-72, 103-104
basic, 70-82
contraindications to, 59, 76
health teaching in, 58-61, 63, 64, 78
reaction to, 60-61, 75
treatment of, 60-61, 75
of refugees, 87-91
health teaching and, 89
surveillance and, 89-92
for retired citizens, 103-104
risk factors and, 49, 58, 76
routine, 70-82
schedules of, 73, 75
screening vaccinee and, 49, 58-61, 76, 90
sequelae of, 66
in U.S.A., 46, 77
see also Vaccination
Immunizations, record keeping and maintaining of, 64, 76, 87, 100
Impetigo, 211-213
bacteria responsible for, 212
primary prevention of, 212-213
symptoms of, 212
transmission of, 212
treatment of, 212
Incidence rate, 5
Infectious hepatitis, see Hepatitis, A
Infectious polyneuritis, 104

Inflammation: definition of, 18
  histamine in process of, 18, 38-39
  leukotaxine in process of, 18
  pus and, 19
Influenza vaccine, 103-104
Interferon, 20
Invading organism, destruction of, 30

Kupffer cells, 17. See also Reticuloendothelial cells
Kwell (Kwellada), 139, 145

Legislative action, 10-12
Leukotaxine, 18
Liver function test (SGOT and SGPT), 121, 125
Lupus erythematosus, 37
Lymph nodes, 21
  antibody formation and, 23
  reticuloendothelial cells and, 17
Lymphocytes, 22, 23
  adaptive, 35
  bursal, 23, 34-35
    origin and location of, 35
  in cellular immunity, 24, 29, 34
  conversion into plasma cells of, 24
  in humoral immunity, 24, 28, 34
  primitive, 35
  processing of, 35
  sensitized, 22, 23, 28, 29
    delayed reaction allergy and, 38-39
    destruction of invading organism by, 30-31
    division of, 29
    release of, 29, 30

  types of organisms destroyed by, 31
  in viral infection, 31
  thymic, 23, 34-35
    origin and location of, 35
Lymphocytic immunity, 22. See also Immunity, adaptive, cellular
Lymphoid tissues, 22
  exposure to antigen, 22
Lysosomes, 19, 38

Macrophages, 18, 19
Malaria, 97-99
  malaria-suppressant drugs, 98, 99
    administration schedule for travelers, 99
  transmission of, 98
Measles, German, see Rubella
Measles, red, 44. See also Rubeola
Metronidazole, 152, 198
  alcohol and, 198
  and contraindications to administration in pregnancy, 198
Microscopy, darkfield, 187-188. See also Syphilis, diagnostic tests for
Monilia, 194-197
  carbohydrate diet and, 196-197
  diagnosis of, 191, 194
    differentiated from syphilis, 194
  fungi responsible for, 194
  health teaching and, 192, 196-197
  incubation period of, 195
  neonatal thrush infection and, 195-196
  in pregnancy, 195-196

and test of cure, 196
recurrence of, 195-196
symptoms of, 192
transmission of, 195
treatment and control of, 195-197
and test of cure, 195
*see also Candida albicans;* Urethritis, nongonococcal
Monocytes, *see* Macrophages
Mononucleosis, infectious, 131-134
diagnosis of, 132
Paul-Bunnell-Davidsohn (PBD) test in, 132
incubation period of, 133
signs and symptoms, 132
transmission of, 133
treatment and control of, 133-134
virus responsible for, 132-133, 178-179
Mumps, 70, 82-83
vaccination for, 82-83
administration schedule of, 82
contraindications to, 82
Myasthenia gravis, 37
*Mycobacterium bovis (M. bovis),* *see* Tuberculosis, organism responsible for
*Mycobacterium tuberculosis (M. tuberculosis), see* Tuberculosis, organism responsible for

*Neisseria gonorrheae (N. gonorrheae),* 172. *See also* Gonorrhea
Neomycin, as allergen, 81, 82

Nurse, role in community health: in control and prevention of:
roundworm infection, 150
sexually transmitted diseases, 168, 174-175, 184, 193
skin diseases, 213, 215
tuberculosis, 240-241, 246, 248
in immunization, 89-92 passim
Nystatin, 195

*Opthalmia neonatorum, see* Chlamydia; Gonorrhea

Parasites: definition of, 137
intestinal, 90-91, 97, 99-100, 146-153
and skin infestations, 138-146
health teaching about, 100, 150
screening refugees for, 90-91, 149, 150, 152
types of, 99, 138, 146
in U.S.A. and Canada, 146, 148-149
*see also* Ascariasis; Enterobiasis; Giardiasis; Pediculosis; Ringworm; Scabies; *Toxocara canis; Toxocara catis;* Toxoplasmosis
Pediculosis, 138-140
areas of infestation, 138, 140
control measures for eradication of outbreaks of, 140
health teaching about, 140
signs of, 138
transmission of, 139

treatment and control of, 139-140

Pelvic inflammatory disease (PID), 170, 199. *See also* Gonorrhea, complications of

Penicillin, 189, 224

Pertusis, 59, 70, 72-75
  vaccination, 74-75, 76
    contraindications to, 76
    reaction to, 76
    secondary complications of, 74
  vaccine, 72-75
    basic, 72-75

Phagocytosis, 26, 28
  opsonization and, 28
  resistance to, 28

Pharynx, lymphoid tissues of, 22

Pinworms, *see* Enterobiasis

Placental barrier, 72, 104-105, 189

Plasma cells, 24-25
  function of, 24-25

Poison invy toxin, 39

Poliomyelitis, 32, 45, 66, 71, 76-78

Poliomyelitis vaccine, 76-78, 89, 92
  administration of, in pregnancy, 77, 104
  administration schedule of, 77
  forms of, 76-77
  sensitivity to, 77
  storage and handling of, 77-78

Polymorphonuclear neutrophils, 18

Prevention, levels of, 5-8, 57, 72
  primary prevention, 5, 7, 57, 72
  secondary prevention, 7-8
  tertiary prevention, 8

Prostatitis, 170. *See also* Gonorrhea, complications of

Psoriasis, 95, 214-215

Public health, and sexually transmitted diseases (STDs), 168

Pus: cleansing from circulation of, 19
  formation of, 19

Respiratory tract, lymphoid tissues of, 22

Reticuloendothelial cells, 26
  digestive enzymes of, 26
  function of, 17
  Kupffer cells, 17
  location of, 17

Reticuloendothelial system (RES), 17, 18, 20, 48

Rheumatic fever, 37

Ringworm, 141-143
  areas of infestation, 143
  athletes' foot and, 141, 142
  diagnosis of, 141, 143
    differential, 141
  organism responsible for, 141
  preventive control measures for, 142
  signs and symptoms of, 141
  transmission of, 142, 143
  treatment of, 142

Roundworms, *see* Ascariasis

Rubella, 45, 49, 70, 78-80
  effect on fetus during pregnancy, 78, 80
  vaccination, 78
    administration schedule of, 78-79
    health teaching about, 78-79, 80
    hemagglutination-inhibition test and, 79-80
    in pregnancy, 78-80, 104

program for women, 79
vaccine, 78-80, 83
Rubeola, 44, 45, 49, 71, 80-82
case report, 44
vaccination, 81-82, 104
reaction to, 81
specific contraindications to,
81-82, 104
tuberculin skin test and, 81-82
vaccine, 80-82, 83

Salmonella, 157-164
diagnosis of, 159-160
staphylococus food poisoning
and, 160
epidemiological measures in
controlling, 162-163
health teaching about, 162, 163
immune response, 159-160
incubation period of, 159, 163
organism responsible for, characteristics of, 159-161
distribution of, 160-161
endotoxin production by, 160
strains of, 160
temperature sensitivity of, 161
as reportable illness, 158
symptoms of, 158-160
transmission of, 159, 161-162
treatment of, 162
*Salmonella paratyphi, see* Salmonella, organism responsible
for, strains of
*Salmonella typhi,* 160. *See also*
Salmonella, organism re-
sponsible for, strains of
*Sarcoptes scabiei* (itch mite), 144.
*See also* Scabies
Scabies, 143-146

diagnosis of, 144
organism responsible for, 144
prodromal period of, 145
signs and symptoms of, 144
transmission of, 144
treatment and control of, 145-
146
Serotonin, 38, 39
Serum glutamic-oxaloabetic transaminase (SGOT), *see* Hepatitis, A, diagnosis of
Serum glutamic-pyrovic transaminase (SGPT), *see* Heptati-
tis, A, diagnosis of
Serum hepatitis, *see* Hepatitis, B
SGOT, *see* Liver function test
SGPT, *see* Liver function test
Shingles, *see* Chickenpox
Skin conditions, noncommunicable,
*see* Acne; Eczema; Psoriasis
Skin infections, *see* Conjunctivitis;
Impetigo
Smallpox, 32, 44, 49, 66, 94-97,
104
vaccination, 95-97, 104
contraindications to, 95-96,
104
health teaching about, 96
pregnancy and, 95-96, 104
reaction to, 96-97
sequelae of, 96-97
vaccine, 94-97
administration schedule of,
94-97
*Staphylococus aureus,* 212. *See
also* Impetigo
Streptococcal infections, 219-225
control of, 225
food processing and, 225

organism responsible for, 223-224

resistance and susceptibility to, 224-225

toxin of, 223-224

types of, 223

*see also Streptococcus pyogenes*

otitis media and, 220-222, 223

characteristics of, 221

hearing impairment and, 221, 223

treatment of, 221-222

primary prevention of, 224

scarlet fever, 222-225

immunity to, 223

signs and symptoms of, 222

secondary sequelae of, 220

tonsillitis and, 220-222

symptoms of, 221

therapy for, 221

transmission of, 224

treatment of, 224

*Streptococcus pyogenes (S. pyogenes)*, 223-225. *See also* Streptococcal infections

Syphilis, 185-191

bacteria responsible for, 188

"flash-freezing" technique and, 188

congenital, 187, 188, 190

diagnosis of, 188

control of, 187, 188-191

contact tracing and, 190

diagnostic tests for, 187-188

dormancy of infection of, 186-187

health teaching and, 190-191

incidence of, 185

incubation period of, 189

"inoculation" sites of, 185

pregnancy and, 187, 189, 190-191

risk factors of, 185

stages of, 185-187

symptoms of, 185-187

transmission of, 188-189

treatment of, 189-190

and test of cure, 189

T-cells, 34-35

Test of cure, 173, 189, 193, 195, 198, 199, 201

Tetanus: bacteria, spores of, 73

health care teaching and, 75

toxin, 21, 26, 32

vaccination, 45, 70, 75-76, 104

case report, 45

reaction to, 75

specific contraindication to, 76

vaccine, basic, 72-76, 89, 92

Tetracycline, 173, 189, 199, 200-201

Throat, lymphoid tissue of, 22

Thymic hormone, 35

Thymus gland, 35

cellular immunity, impairment of, 35

role of, 35

Tissue histocytes, *see* Macrophages

Tissue repair, role of fibroblasts in, 19

Toxins, destruction of, 20

*Toxocara canis,* 152-153

*Toxocara cati,* 152-153

Toxoplasmosis, 152

in pregnancy, 152

Travel, *see* Immunization, overseas travel

*Treponema pallidum (T. pallidum)*, 188. *See also* Syphilis, bacteria responsible for
Trichomonas, 197-198
  diagnosis of, 191, 197
  dormancy of, 197
  health teaching and, 198
  incubation period of, 197
  recurrence of, 197-198
  symptoms of, 192, 197
  transmission of, 197-198
  treatment and control of, 198
  and test of cure, 198
*Trichomonas vaginalis,* 171, 197-198. *See also* Urethritis, nongonococcal; Vaginitis
Tuberculosis (TB), 31, 101, 102, 228
  bacille Calmette-Guérin (BCG) vaccination against, 102, 237, 246-248
  bovine, 235
  control of, 234, 237, 241-248
    prophylactic program and, 245
    screening programs for, 242-248
  diagnosis of, 232, 234-235
    culture of bacillus from sputum test and, 234
    microscopy test of smear of sputum and, 234
  health teaching and, 237, 240-241
  implantation sites of, 230-231
  initial infection in, 230-231, 232, 234
  immune response to, 231
  latency of, 234
  mantoux, 59, 102, 232, 234, 242-246

    minimum negative measurements and, 243
    mumps immunization and, 82
    rubeola immunization and, 81-82
    specific contraindications to, 244
  organism responsible for, 235, 236
    atypical mycobacteria differentiated from, 235
    staining of, 235
  PPD test, *see* Tuberculosis, mantoux
  prevention of, 237, 241-248
  progressive, 231-232
    cavity formation and, 231-232
  signs and symptoms of, 232, 234
  stages of, 230-233
  transmission of, 229, 236-237
  treatment of, 238, 239-240
    drug programs and, 239-240
  tuberculin skin test, Tuberculosis, mantoux
Typhoid vaccine, 94, 101-102

Urethritis, 169-170, 197, 199, 200, 201
  nongonococcal (NGU), 171, 197, 199
  *see also* Chlamydia; Gonorrhea
Urticaria, 40, 61-62

Vaccination, 21, 32
  adaptive immunity and, 32
  attenuation of live organisms and, 32
  methods of, 66
  pregnancy and, 60, 104-105

responses to, 32-33, 48, 72
schedules and factors influenc-
ing, 71, 73
Vaccine, 33
abnormalities of, 65
absorbed, 48, 72
adjuvant (depot) effect, 49, 72
administration of, 66
administration of, 65-66
antigenic quality of, 48
basic, 71-82
booster dose of, 33, 48
combined, 72-82
immune response to, 72
MMR (measles, mumps, and
rubella), 72, 83
contraindicated in pregnancy,
104-105
efficacy of, 71-72
influenza, 103, 105
contraindications to administration of, 103
and Guillaine-Barré syndrome,
104
live, and tuberculin sensitivity, 59
paratyphoid A and B, *see* Vaccine, typhoid
primary, *see* Vaccine, basic
TAB, *see* Vaccine, typhoid
TABT, *see* Vaccine, typhoid
types of, 48
typhoid, 94, 101-102, 104
administration schedule of,
101-102
Vaccines, combining of, 71-72
Vaginitis, 169, 191-202
health history and, 191
health teaching and, 192-193
intrauterine device (IUD), and,
191-192
nonsexually transmitted, 193,
194-197
acid-alkaline balance of vagina
and, 193-194
Döderlein's bacilli and, 193,
200
estrogen release and, 193-
194
*see also* Monilia
nonspecific, 200-201
coexistance with other STDs,
201
diagnostic test of, 200
sexually transmitted, 194, 197-
202. *See also* Chlamydia;
Trichomonas; Vaginitis,
nonspecific
symptoms of, 192
Varicella zoster virus, 115, 178-
179
dormancy of, 115
virulence of, 114
*see also* Chickenpox
Venereal disease research laboratory (VDRL) test, 187,
190-191. *See also* Syphilis,
diagnostic tests for
Viruses: definition of, 179
mechanism of development and
release of, 179

Whooping cough, *see* Pertusis
Wood's light, 143. *See also* Ringworm, diagnosis of
World Health Organization (WHO),
44, 94

Yellow fever, 32, 94

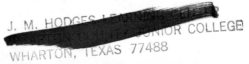